Nursing Interventions
in Depression

Nursing Interventions in Depression

Edited by

Carol A. Rogers, M.N., R.N.

Clinical Specialist
Psychiatric/Mental Health Nursing
College of Nursing
Rush University
Chicago, Illinois

Jane Ulsafer-Van Lanen, M.S., R.N.

Assistant Professor/Associate Chairperson
Department of Psychiatric Nursing
College of Nursing
Rush University
Chicago, Illinois

 Grune & Stratton, Inc.
(Harcourt Brace Jovanovich, Publishers)
Orlando   San Diego   New York
London   Toronto   Montreal   Sydney   Tokyo

Library of Congress Cataloging in Publication Data

Main entry under title:

Nursing interventions in depression.

Includes bibliographies and index.
1. Depression, Mental—Nursing. 2. Psychiatric
nursing. I. Rogers, Carol A. II. Ulsafer-Van Lanen,
Jane. [DNLM: 1. Depressive Disorder—nursing.
WM 171 N974]
RC537.N87   1985   616.85′27   85-5485
ISBN 0-8089-1710-2

Grune & Stratton, Inc.
Orlando, FL 32887

Distributed in the United Kingdom by
Grune & Stratton, Ltd.
24/28 Oval Road, London NW 1

Library of Congress Catalog Number   85-5485
International Standard Book Number   0-8089-1710-2

Printed in the United States of America
85 86 87 88 10 9 8 7 6 5 4 3 2 1

To our daughters Beth and Kathleen, who finished their gestations concurrently with the book's completion.

Contents

Preface

The material for *Nursing Interventions in Depression* grew out of the Fifth Annual Psychiatric Nursing Symposium sponsored by the Department of Psychiatric Nursing at Rush-Presbyterian–St. Luke's Medical Center, Chicago, Illinois. Our aim then was to present psychiatric nursing interventions and developing protocols that had been used successfully in both our practice and our teaching. We have attempted to remain true to this purpose in the preparation of this book. Because of the diversity of contributors, we are able to represent the treatment of persons with affective disorders in a variety of age groups and treatment settings. In addition, the book raises some critical concerns about the direction of psychiatric nursing practice and education.

It is our hope that the material presented here will enhance understanding, and support the use of new or different interventions. We were stimulated by the dearth of topic-specific references for nurses wishing to incorporate contemporary theory and research in their practice. Encouragement came from the responses of our colleagues in various practice settings. Many others also assisted us, and we wish to express our appreciation to them. In particular, we acknowledge the contributors to this book, we could not approach their level of expertise in preparing the diverse material. Thanks also to family, friends, and typists, who assisted in so many ways. Finally, our deepest appreciation goes to the numerous women and men with affective disorders who have been recipients of our care. Their "getting better" encouraged us to continue our efforts to grow, and develop improved intervention methods.

Contributors

Susan S. Anderson, M.S.N., R.N., C.S.
Instructor/Unit Leader
Department of Psychiatric Nursing
Rush-Presbyterian–St. Luke's Medical Center
Sheridan Road Hospital
Chicago, Illinois

Rosalind D. Cartwright, Ph.D.
Chairperson, Psychology and Social Sciences
Director, Sleep Disorder Service
    and Research Center
Rush-Presbyterian–St. Luke's Medical Center
Chicago, Illinois

Kathryn Gleason Cook, M.A., M.S., R.N.
Assistant Professor
Department of Psychiatric Nursing
College of Nursing
Rush University
Chicago, Illinois

Kathleen Ryan Delaney, D.N.Sc., R.N.
Chicago Lake Shore Hospital
Chicago, Illinois

David Duda, M.S., R.N.
Instructor/Unit Leader
Department of Psychiatric Nursing
College of Nursing
Rush University
Rush-Presbyterian–St. Luke's Medical Center
Chicago, Illinois

Jan Fawcett, M.D.

Professor and Chairperson
Department of Psychiatry
Rush-Presbyterian–St. Luke's Medical Center
Chicago, Illinois

Marian Fiske, M.S.N., R.N.

Assistant Professor/Associate Chairperson
Department of Psychiatric Nursing
College of Nursing
Rush University
Chicago, Illinois

Howard M. Kravitz, D.O.

Assistant Professor
Departments of Psychiatry, Psychology and Social Sciences
Medical Director, Sleep Disorder Service
    and Research Center
Rush-Presbyterian–St. Luke's Medical Center
Chicago, Illinois

Priscilla Lynch, M.S., R.N.

Practitioner–Teacher
Psychiatric/Medical Liaison
Assistant Professor
College of Nursing
Rush University
Chicago, Illinois

Dennis A. Nakanishi, B.S.

Department of Psychiatric Nursing
Rush-Presbyterian–St. Luke's Medical Center
Chicago, Illinois

Paula F. Price, M.S., R.N.

Captain, U.S. Army Nurse Corps
Bayne-Jones Community Hospital
Fort Polk, Louisiana

Carol A. Rogers, M.N., R.N.
Clinical Specialist
Psychiatric/Mental Health Nursing
College of Nursing
Rush University
Chicago, Illinois

Katherine Y. Sasaki, M.S., R.N.
Clinical Specialist
Fresno State University
Fresno, California

Debra Sivesind, M.S.N., R.N.
Instructor/Unit Leader
College of Nursing
Department of Psychiatric Nursing
Rush-Presbyterian–St. Luke's Medical Center
Chicago, Illinois

Marsha D. Snyder, M.S.N., R.N.
Assistant Professor–Unit Leader
Department of Psychiatric Nursing
College of Nursing
Rush University
Chicago, Illinois

Marietta Nolan Stevens, M.N., R.N.
Instructor/Practitioner–Teacher
Department of Psychiatric Nursing
College of Nursing
Rush University
Chicago, Illinois

Jane Ulsafer-Van Lanen, M.S., R.N.
Assistant Professor/Associate Chairperson
Department of Psychiatric Nursing
College of Nursing
Rush University
Chicago, Illinois

1

Reconciling Models of Depression

Carol A. Rogers

Acceptance of an ideological view of mental illness that involves a choice between personality, biology, or environment, is representative of much of contemporary treatment in mental health care. These ideological models separate mind and body, and sustain artificial boundaries among disciplines and their knowledge bases while inhibiting the application of new knowledge to patient care. Research now implicates personality, biology, and environment in the etiology and maintenance of affective disorders. In the fields of biochemistry and neurophysiology, such research has led to significant progress in the identification, differentiation, and treatment of depression and mania. Concurrently, studies in the behavioral sciences are elucidating the formative or mediating role of psychological and sociological variables in the onset and maintenance of these disorders.

Reliance on conceptual frameworks that disregard data derived from current research on affective disorders reduces treatment efficacy. The dominant models guiding psychiatric nursing practice are psychodynamic and psychosocial in nature. Within these frameworks, new knowledge concerning biological variables is often not utilized. In some instances, biological theories are considered antithetical to psychiatric nursing practice. If models are considered reflections of the state of science at a particular time, which continue to change or evolve as the present state of knowledge expands, then currently articulated psychodynamic or psychosocial frameworks taught and used by psychiatric nurses are limited in application and fall short as scientific models of practice.

At issue in this discussion is whether or not existing psychiatric nursing frameworks adequately conceptualize the phenomena of interest to our practice. For purposes of this chapter, the phenomena of interest are behavioral responses to the affective disorders (depression and mania). Theories regarding the specific relations among variables thought to effect, cause, or contribute to these behavioral responses arise from the conceptual model. A psychosocial model identifies constructs and propositions that refer to psychological and social processes thought to explain or influence responses to illness. From this viewpoint, biologic factors are excluded. In light of current advances in knowledge regarding affective disorders, treating depression from this framework becomes analogous to treating a diabetic crisis in purely behavioral terms and ignoring the physiological disturbance.

We can ask ourselves these questions:

- Can psychiatric nursing afford to treat neurophysiological and biochemical theories as irrelevant to the treatment of behavioral responses of affective disorders?
- Is the increasing knowledge regarding the relationship between brain and behavior not useful in assessment and intervention?
- Can we continue to teach our students that the vegetative signs of a depression are either maladaptive or signs of manipulation?
- Can the standard intervention for depression continue to be supported in the face of growing evidence for the heterogeneity of depression?

The literal intention to exclude biologic determinants and concomitants in nursing approaches to affective disorders may not exist, and yet, the identification of psychiatric nursing with interpersonal, intrapersonal, and system variables alone has resulted in this exclusion. Fagin (1981) argues that psychiatric nursing adopted a medical model approach to psychiatric care, namely psychotherapy, that contributed to our current tenuous status. This chapter takes the similar position that the accent on psychotherapeutic intervention alone has gained us little and may have cost us much. Among her recommendations for treating our troubled status, Fagin proposes the development of other conceptual models for practice. Mitsunaga (1982) agrees with the proposal and suggests such strategies as incorporating primary care into the undergraduate nursing experience, which should broaden the view of the functions besides psychotherapy that are germane to our practice.

THE NEED FOR OTHER CONCEPTUAL MODELS OF DEPRESSION

The premise of this chapter supports the aims of nursing leaders concerning the need for other conceptual models for psychiatric nursing practice. This can be accomplished by widening the knowledge base from which we borrow and adapt concepts and theories to explain and guide our practice. All new research findings pertinent to affective disorders can be investigated for applicability to our practice. Exclusion of data will then be based on nonadaptability to psychiatric nursing management of illness, rather than on the basis of ideologic definitions or interdisciplinary rivalries.

Several events have converged to shape the present problem.

1. Increasing acuity and severity of primary depressive illnesses.
2. Improvements in identification and classification of depressive states.
3. Major advances in knowledge of etiology and treatment of affective disorders.

The Increasing Acuity and Severity of Primary Depressive Illness

Few practitioners can deny the occurrence of the first event. Clinical observations of patient populations utilizing hospitals and clinics bear out this finding: individuals presenting for treatment, either voluntarily or involuntarily, are more often in acute stages of illness and exhibit symptomatology of severe proportions. These individuals are suicidal, uncontrollable, or so incapacitated that initial treatment measures involve assistance with basic functions of eating, sleeping, and providing safety. Estimates of the range of depressive symptomology, from depressive in nature (grief reactions and other situational responses) to serious psychopathology, report 15% of the population having difficulty in managing life problems and 3% of these having serious primary disease (Katz, 1980). Whether this 3% represents an actual increase in numbers of persons with severe affective illness, increased utilization of mental health care facilities by the severely ill, or reflects the effects of improvements in diagnostic criteria, the empirical evidence reveals a treatment population that has grown more seriously ill.

For psychiatric nursing, the existence of greater numbers of severely ill individuals in the treatment population necessitates a shift in emphasis from a primarily interactional, behavioral focus to one that accounts for physiologic dysfunction as well. This shift challenges our knowledge and skills while also challenging some basic assumptions or beliefs regarding illness states and appropriate patient responses to them. For instance, in the acute and severe states of depression, in which suicidal or melancholic feelings and behaviours are prominent, the individual suffers from "serious somatic dysregulation" and is "simply too ill to derive benefit from verbal therapies alone" (Akiskal, 1979). Somatic interventions, based on needs for nutrition, safety, and rest become the priority in order to restore the individual to a state in which he or she can respond to interpersonal interventions. At this point, the psychosocial perspective assesses such responses as isolation, apathy, and lack of interest in surroundings as maladaptive responses to one's environment. This necessitates interventions, based on interpersonal reinforcement theory, that encourage activity, task performance, and contact with others. The addition of neurophysiologic theory, hypothesizing that these anhedonic behaviors of severe depression prevent learning by reinforcement, modifies initial assessments and interventions. What first appear as maladaptive responses to the environment are reconstructed as biological dysfunction. From this perspective, interventions focused on activity, performance, and social contact for the patient appear counterproductive and premature at best, and inhumane and painful at worst. Initial interventions such as acceptance of behaviors associated with severe depression as adaptive and support in the form of safety, rest, hydration, reassurance, and active listening are missing. Theories regarding the etiology of this biologic dysfunction need not be an issue since experimental studies indicate that the clinical picture of severe depression is the same whether the precipitant is object loss, environmental stressors, genetic predisposition, or neuroamine deficit.

Use of self as a therapeutic tool is essential, as knowledge regarding establishment of trust along with communication strategies enhances the restorative aims of this stage of treatment. What has been added is information about and recognition of new and viable information regarding physiologic dysruption of usual functioning. This physiologic dysruption influences cognitive and motor functioning as well as vegetative and emotional functioning (Beck, 1967). Once basic life-maintenance processes have been restored, cognitive and motor dysfunction may remain. This suggests that intervention strategies should encompass conceptualizations of depression and mania as the results of biochemical and psychological stresses. Thus, knowledge of the relations between behavior and brain functioning become necessary components for understanding the behavioral responses of affective disorders.

Improvements in Identification and Classification of Depressive States

The lack of precise definitions for depression and mania has been a source of confusion and criticism among clinicians and researchers. The proliferation of meanings of these terms without attempts to distinguish between clinical depression and forms of unhappiness has been a chief obstacle to effective treatment of these disorders. Criticism from psychiatric nurses has focused on the medical model approach associated with the standard classification scheme, the Diagnostic and Statistical Manual II (DSM-II). This often resulted in persons being labelled according to such characteristics as social class or gender, or in a fashion that reflected the practitioners' particular philosophy of treatment (Williams & Wilson, 1982). While such criticisms are warranted, they apparently led psychiatric nurses to identify only those particular aspects of depression thought to be amenable to psychiatric nursing intervention. Again, these decisions were made on the basis of accepted frameworks of care that guided choice of phenomena of concern as well as understanding of illness states. Unfortunately, advances in the understanding of etiology and maintenance of depression and in the classification of this disorder (including mania) have made many conventional psychiatric nursing conceptualizations of affective illness states outmoded, limited, and inadequate for assessment and intervention in treating a population that is ill or at risk. The conventional psychiatric nursing conceptualization of depression, reflected in most basic texts and articles, teaches that depression is a grief reaction or situational response resulting from either psychological or social stressors or both.* From this, interventions are aimed at interpersonal and intrapersonal resolution of stressors. Little information is provided on clinical manifestations, etiology, and management issues and approaches of primary depression or melancholia. Yet, the development of Diagnostic and Statistical Manual III (DSM-III) (American Psychiatric Association, 1980) has provided clarity and consensus about the description of the illness state called depression. It has also provoked debate over treatment issues and approaches that providers of mental health services cannot ignore.

For psychiatric nurses, as clinicians and teachers, the meaning of the term depression as currently understood is more than a grief reaction or situational response to stress. While these remain important types of depressions, other types, representing more serious disease and disruption in an individual and his or her family, are also prevalent and require treatment. Using a multiaxial framework, the behaviors, characteristics, and expected impairments common to different types of depression have been identified and are now classified in the DSM-III. This phenomenologic approach calls upon the genetic, biological, psychological, and environmental evidence thus far accumulated. By eschewing a theoretical approach, practitioners can agree on what they see. As a result, theoretical differences, based not on separate and distinct conceptualizations of illness but on separate and distinct conceptualizations of phenomena of concern, guide treatment approaches. Recognition of the DSM-III as a valid, reliable means of assessment and planning for interventions for depressed patients, can be given by psychiatric nurses without compromising patient-centered concerns. This is due to its reliance on descriptive, phenomenologic criteria for assessment that avoids theoretical (etiologic) frameworks as a basis for diagnosis (Williams & Wilson, 1982). Thus psychiatric nursing, will link care-giving to distinctions in phenomena of concern and domain of practice rather than linking assessment and intervention to conceptual approaches that rely on limited explanations of the illness state.

---

*Some recent exceptions are texts by: Stuart and Sundeen (1983) and Pasquali, et al. (1981).

Major Advances in Knowledge of Etiology and Treatment of Affective Disorders

The third event that has led to questions regarding the relevance of purely psychosocial frameworks for psychiatric nurses has been the major advances in knowledge regarding the etiology and treatment of affective disorders. Some mention has already been made of psychobiologic theories. While these have been the most visible scientific advances, developments in psychological and sociological theory concerning factors that maintain or assist in formation of depression also must be considered. This becomes especially true with the realization that much of the work in these latter fields concentrates on female depressed populations who constitute the majority of ill persons as well as the majority of persons at risk (Weissman & Klerman, 1977).

Some may disregard or discount the biology of depressions as being reductionistic (Peele, 1981), but such strict distinction among fields of science is "heuristically sterile" (Akiskal, 1979) and is unworthy of the aims of psychiatric nursing practice. Rather than thinking of biological determinants as reductionistic, which suggests that all behavior is determined strictly by nervous system functioning, many scientists and practitioners now consider biological determinants to be part of the "interaction between life events and neurobiology in the genesis of depressive disorders" (Akiskal, 1979. See also Stuart & Sundeen, 1983; Pasquali et al., 1981).

BIOCHEMICAL THEORIES OF AFFECTIVE DISORDERS

Biological explanations of behavior are a relatively new phenomena. Although the roots can be traced to the 1950s with the discovery of drugs that could alleviate some of the symptoms of mental illness, real interest in tracing the biochemical changes associated with drug action is recent. Coupled with sound scientific methodology, this interest has led to new insights about the biochemical mechanisms of mental illness, especially depression and mania. Most psychiatric nurses are familiar with biochemical theories of affective disorders as they relate to the role of such neurotransmitters as dopamine, serotonin, and norepinephrine in controlling or effecting behavior. Because of the many inconsistencies in the monoamine theory of depression (Mendels & Frazer, 1974), theoretical development has taken new directions. The simplistic model of shortages and surpluses of a single neurotransmitter has been replaced by new lines of investigation suggesting that there are different biochemical types of depression (Schildkraut, 1965). Maas (1975) classified two types of depression, based on hypothetical differences in monoaminergic mechanisms. These were labelled *Type A* and *Type B* depressions; each was distinguished by differences in pretreatment level of urinary 3-methoxy-4-hydroxyphenylethelene glycol (MHPG), response to a stimulant challenge test with dextroamphetamine, and response to the tricyclic antidepressants amitriptyline and imipramine (Akiskal, 1979). Deficits in norepinephrine were responsible for Type A depressions and deficits in serotonin were responsible for Type B depressions. Still more recent clinical studies have challenged this norepinephrine–serotonin dichotomy while supporting the notion of biochemically heterogeneous depressions (Sabelli et al., 1983).

This very brief introduction to biologic explanations of affective disorders is meant to illustrate the advances made thus far in theory formation as well as in clinical treatment. It is well known that biochemical treatment of affective disorders, regardless of whether or not the person is hospitalized, remains a significant problem due to the differences in individual response to antidepressant medication, subjective selection of drug by the psychiatrist, and the state of knowledge (Stern et al., 1980). Often, the lag between theory development and its application is unreasonably long. Fortunately, because much of the biochemical research is tied to clinical trials, benefits accrue to the ill individual as well as to the knowledge base. For a comprehensive review of biological contributions to the assessment and treatment of affective disorders, the reader is referred to Chapters 2 and 5.

Genetic Factors as Significant Determinants of Mental Illness

The contribution of heredity to the development of mental disorders is of interest to researchers and laypersons alike. The idea that genetic factors are significant determinants of vulnerability to mental illness has found reluctant acceptance among mental health professionals (Gershon, 1980), and yet genetic research has made valuable contributions toward understanding depression and mania, especially. It was the search for a genetic factor in the etiology of depression that led to the separation of bipolar from unipolar illness states (Winokur et al., 1969). Evidence for the genetic hypothesis has come from four sources: (1) family studies comparing affective illness rates between and within generations (Winokur & Cadoret, 1977; Bunney, 1981); (2) twin studies comparing affective illness rates between monozygotic and dizygotic twins (Allen, 1976; Bertelson et al., 1977); (3) cross-rearing studies; and (4) linkage studies using genetic markers to trace other traits through several generations or in siblings (Weissman & Klerman, 1977). The family and twin studies have produced the most evidence for a genetic factor in affective illness. The initial report from The Yale University–National Institute of Mental Health Collaborative Family Study of Depression presents the "first substantive collaborative results of the overall risk of various psychiatric disorders . . . among first degree relatives of the four proband groups" (Weissman et al., 1984). Being one of the few studies to employ control groups of "never-ill" persons, the Yale study concludes that "major depression had the highest frequency (of occurence) in the relatives of all groups of affectively ill persons" (major depression and bipolar-I illnesses). Such studies have implications for differential diagnosis, case-finding, treatment planning, and possibly, prevention.

Nonbiological Factors Causing Depression

Evidence linking depressive symptomology with factors other than biologic ones has been accumulating for years. In fact, the belief that depression is psychogenic in origin had predominated psychiatric treatment until recently. To this end, many psychological models have been created to explain the etiology of depression. From the Freudian interpretation of depression as anger turned inward, to the contemporary formulation of Beck (1967), which emphasizes cognitive analysis of depressive thoughts and beliefs, psychodynamic models have dominated the understanding and threatment of depression. Additionally, sociological factors such as marital status (Gove, 1972), availability of other support systems (Warheit, 1979) and number of undesirable life events (Paykel, 1976; Petrich & Holmes, 1981) have been identified as "formative" in the onset of depressive illness. The research findings on psychosocial and other environmental factors are voluminous and widely published. From this material, the author has chosen data representing psychological and sociological findings to illustrate the relationship of nonbiologic factors and depression.

"A frequent observation in epidemiologic studies of depression is that women preponderate" (Weissman & Klerman, 1977). This difference in rates of depression between the sexes is a clinically observable phenomenon for which there have been various biological, genetic, and sociocultural explanations. Biologic formulations have attempted to correlate mood changes with endocrine imbalances occurring premenstrually, during menopause, and during the postpartum period. Genetic studies have investigated X-linkage transmission as the basis of sex differences. Most formulations have lost favor due to insufficient or mixed findings and the current cultural climate that "disapproves of biologically based explanations for . . . distinctions between males and females" (Peele, 1981). Several models relating social causes to the observed sex-linked psychological differences have been developed. The learned helplessness model of Seligman (1974) is perhaps the most striking, as it is founded on animal experiments that have been replicated in special situations with human subjects. The model extrapolates from the discovery that animals, having learned through repeated trials of their inability to control the experience of noxious stimuli, respond passively by giving up and withdrawing (Seligman, 1974). The parallels between these responses and those of depressed humans (especially women) led to the formulation that a negative appraisal of ability to influence the environment can result in depressive illness. This behavioral state (called *learned help-*

lessness) is characterized by impairment in adaptive functioning and feelings of helplessness and powerlessness. This model is thought to have special relevance to women as it reflects the effects of social conditioning and sex-role stereotypes in Western cultures.

The second set of nonbiologic factors considered relevant in the etiology and maintenance of depression involve the study of life events. These studies call attention to a limitation in most biologic explanations of depression, i.e., a disregard for the influence of the unavoidable events and stresses of living. Literature on life stress and illness has confirmed a link between clusters of events causing disruption in living patterns and onset of disease (Hawkins et al., 1957; Rahe et al., 1964). From this perspective, a variety of psychiatric illnesses have been studied and also found to be linked to life stress. Investigations by Paykel (1974) and Brown and Harris (1978) of number of life events and type of psychiatric illness experienced, revealed that suicide attempts and depression are preceded by the highest concentrations of negative life events. These concentrations were significatly higher than those for the general population.

In addition to higher concentrations, the subjective quality of life events was found to be significantly discriminating for depressive illness (Paykel, 1976). Suicide attempts and depressions were preceded by life events appraised by the patients as threatening, undesirable, and outside their ability to control (Thomson & Hendrie, 1972; Uhlenhuth & Paykel, 1973). Such events as arguments with spouse, marital separation, change to a new type of work, and serious illness or death of a family member were frequent reports. Conflict with spouse was found 15 times more frequently in the history of depressed persons than in that of controls (Petrich & Holmes, 1981). Thus, events reflecting psychosocial theories of depression of loss, blows to self-esteem, and the appraisal of threat figure prominently as antecedants of clinical depression (Paykel, 1976).

Given that life events precede the onset of many depressions, can they be considered causative? What is the impact of those life events experienced as threat or loss on the development of behaviors called depression? Skeptics of life events research point out methodologic problems, such as attenuation and distortion of recall, that raise questions on the likelihood of a significant relationship between life events and depression. Attempts to resolve this question have resulted in recent hypotheses that describe life events as "formative" in the genesis of depression (Paykel, 1979). A certain collection of life events alone does not cause a depressive disorder. Rather, a host of factors relating to the individual and the environment modify the effect of life events to increase or decrease the risk. Some of these modifying factors are social, such as presence or absence of a confidante and extended family, class, early loss of a mother, and unemployment (Warheit, 1979). Others are genetic vulnerability, coping repertoire, and personality traits. The conclusion concerning the relationship of life events to onset of depression is that "life events take their place as one of many factors in multifactorial causation of depressive disorders" (Paykel, 1979).

SUMMARY

The conclusion that there are multiple causative factors responsible for the onset of depression represents a new trend among researchers studying affective disorders. This trend acknowledges the accumulating evidence that unidirectional or single set hypotheses of illness are no longer considered to be satisfactory explanations of depression. Such ideological formulations, still prevalent among psychiatric practitioners, have serious theoretical deficiencies. The major problem is their almost exclusive emphasis on a single set of variables, either biologic, psychologic, or sociologic. This emphasis excludes consideration of other factors found to be causative. Findings from the physical and behavioral sciences as well as from treatment outcome studies, suggest an interdependent relationship among personality, biologic, and environmental factors in the etiology and maintenance of depression. Attempts at reconciling these diverse findings have been sporadic and incomplete. A more comprehensive model, from the viewpoint of number of factors accounted for, is that of Akiskal and McKinney (1975). This model conceptualizes depressive illness as the "feedback interaction of three sets of variables at chemical, experiential and behavioral levels with the diencephalon serving as the field of action." A dysfunction or imbalance on one level is thought to affect the other two. Thus, impairment in any of the three variables can cause a depression. Clinical features may appear similar no matter what combination of variables are involved because all processes converge in a final common pathway in the diencephalon. This unified model accounts for a variety of causative factors—genetic, social or biological—and emphasizes the assessment of patient behaviors (Stuart & Sundeen, 1983).

Specification of causal models will continue. Whether a comprehensive framework for understanding psychopathology will ever be developed remains speculative at present. More importantly, the need to treat populations of psychiatrically ill persons and to identify persons at risk is ever-present. The evidence suggesting interdependent relations among biological, psychological, and sociological factors in the development of affective disorders can be utilized now.

This chapter has identified three events in the mental health care field that call into question current psychosocial models of psychiatric nursing practice. Nursing leaders also have begun to question which models should comprise the accepted framework from which to practice. The concern is not whether psychosocial frameworks are viable models but whether, by themselves, they are inadequate to explain or describe severe types of psychiatric disorder and delineate the full range of human response to affective disorders requiring intervention. Adopting models that are biopsychosocial in nature will enhance the development of the "helping relationship" that is considered the core of the psychiatric nursing specialty. Through this holistic approach, so long espoused by psychiatric nurses, a commitment can be made to cognitive openness rather than idealogic steadfastness, thereby contributing to the advances in treatment of affective disorders through nursing practice and research.

REFERENCES

Akiskal, H. G. (1979). A behavioral approach to depression. In R. A. Dupre (Ed.), *The psychobiology of the depressive disorders: Implications for the effects of stress* (pp. 409–437). New York: Academic Press, Inc.

Akiskal, H. G., & McKinney, W. T., Jr. (1975). Overview of recent research in depression: Integration of ten conceptual models into a comprehensive clinical frame. *Archives of general psychiatry, 32,* 285–305.

Allen, M. G. (1976). Twin studies of affective illness. *Archives of General Psychiatry, 33,* 409–437.

American Psychiatric Association (1980). *Diagnostic and statistical manual of mental disorders* (3rd ed.). Washington, D.C.: The American Psychiatric Association.

Beck, A. T. (1967). *Depression: Cases and treatment.* Philadelphia: University of Pennsylvania Press.

Bertelson, A., Harvald, R., & Hauge, M. (1977). A Danish twin study of manic-depressive disorder. *British Journal of Psychiatry, 130,* 330–351.

Brown, G. W., & Harris, T. (1978). *Social origins of depression: A study of psychiatric disorders in women* (pp. 117–129). London: Tavistock Publications.

Bunney, W. E. (1981). Psychobiological research in manic-depressive illness. In T. A. Ban, R. Gonzalez, A. S. Jablensky, N. A. Satorius, & F. E. Vortanian, *Prevention and Treatment of Depression* (pp. 121–132). Baltimore: University Park Press.

Fagin, C. M. (1981). Psychiatric nursing at the crossroads: Quo vadis. *Perspectives in Psychiatric Care, 19*(3&4), 99–106.

Gershon, E. S. (1980). Genetic factors from a clinical perspective. In J. Mendels & J. D. Amsterdam (Eds.), *Psychobiology of affective disorders: Pfizer symposium on depression* (pp. 25–39). Basel, New York: Karger.

Gove, W. R. (1972). The relationship between sex roles, marital status, and mental illness. *Social Forces, 51,* 34–44.

Hawkins, N. G., Davies, R. & Holmes, T. H. (1957). Evidence of psychosocial factors in pulmonary tuberculosos." *American Review of Tuberculosis Pulmonary Disease, 75,* 768–780.

Katz, M. M. (1980). Depression: A national health problem. In J. Mendels & J. D. Amsterdam (Eds.), *Psychobiology of Affective Disorders: Pfizer Symposium on Depression* (pp. 1–10). Basel, New York: Karger.

Maas, J. W. (1975). Biogenic amines and depression. *Archives of General Psychiatry, 32,* 1357–1361.

Mendels, J. & Frazer, A. (1974). "Brain biogenic amine depletion and mood." *Archives of General Psychiatry, 30,* 447–451.

Mitsunaga, B. K. (1982). "Designing psychiatric/mental health nursing for the future: Problems and prospects." *Journal of Psychiatric Nursing and Mental Health Services, 20*(2), 15–21.

Pasquali, E. A., Alesi, E. G., Arnold, H. M. & DeBasio, N. (1981). *Mental health nursing: A bio-psycho-cultural approach* (pp. 401–410), St. Louis, Toronto, London: The C. V. Mosby Company.

Paykel, E. S. (1974). Recent life events and clinical depression. In E. L. Gunderson & R. H. Rahe (Eds.), *Life Stress and Illness* (pp. 134–163). Springfield, Ill.: Charles C. Thomas.

Paykel, E. S. (1976). Life stress, depression and attempted suicide. *Journal of Human Stress, 2*(3), 3–12.

Paykel, E. S. (1979). Causal relationships between clinical depression and life events. In J. E. Barrett (Ed.), American Psychopathological Association Series, *Stress and mental disorder,* (pp. 71–86) New York: Raven Press.

Peele, S. (1981). Reductionism in the psychology of the eighties: Can biochemistry eliminate addiction, mental illness, and pain? *American Psychologist, 36*(8), 807–818.

Petrich, J. M. & Holmes, T. H. (1981). Recent life events and psychiatric illness. *Psychiatric Annals. 11*(6), 207–218.

Rahe, R. H., Meyer, M., Smith, M., Kjaer, G. & Holmes, T. H. (1964). Social stress and illness onset. *Journal of Psychosomatic Research, 8,* 35–44.

Sabelli, H. C., Fawcett, J., Javaid, J. & Bagri, S. (1983). The methylphenidate test for differentiating desipramine-responsive from nortriptyline-responsive depression. *American Journal of Psychiatry, 140*(2), 212–214.

Schildkraut, J. (1965). Catecholamine hypothesis of affective disorders. *American Journal of Psychiatry, 122,* 509–522.

Seligman, M. E. (1974). Depression and learned helplessness. In R. J. Friedman and M. M. Katz (Eds.), *The psychology of depression: Contemporary theory and research* (pp. 83–113). Washington, D.C.: V. H. Winston & Sons.

Stern, S. L., Rush, A. J. & Mendels, J. (1980). Toward a rational pharmacotherapy of depression. *American Journal of Psychiatry, 137*(5), 545–552.

Stuart, G. W. & Sundeen, S. J. (1983). *Principles and practice of psychiatric nursing* (2nd ed.). St. Louis: The C. V. Mosby Company.

Thomson, J. C. & Hendrie, H. C. (1972). Environmental stress in primary depressive illness. *Archives of General Psychiatry, 26,* 130–132.

Uhlenhuth, E. H. & Paykel, E. S. (1973). Symptom configuration and life events. *American Journal of Psychiatry, 28,* 744–748.

Warheit, G. J. (1979). Life events, coping, stress, and depressive symptomatology. *American Journal of Psychiatry, 136*(4B), 502–507.

Weissman, M. M. & Klerman, G. L. (1977). Sex differences and the epidemiology of depression. *Archives of General Psychiatry, 34,* 98–111.

Weissman, M. M., Gershon, E. S., Kidd, K. K., Prusoff, B. A., Leckman, J. F., Dibble, E., Harmovit, J., Thompson, W. D., Pauls, D. L. & Guroff, J. J. (1984). Psychiatric disorders in the relatives of probands with affective disorders. *Archives of General Psychiatry, 44*(1), 13–21.

Winokur, G. & Cadoret, R. (1977). Genetic studies in depressive disorders. In G. D. Burrows (Ed.), *Handbook of studies in depression,* (pp. 69–77). New York: Excerpta Medica.

Winokur, G., Clayton, P. J. & Reich, T. (1969). *Manic Depressive Illness.* St. Louis: The C. V. Mosby Co.

Williams, J. B. W. and Wilson, H. S. (1982). A Psychiatric Nursing Perspective on DSM-III. *Journal of Psychiatric Nursing and Mental Health Services, 20*(4):14–20.

2

Current Research in Affective Illness

Jan Fawcett
Howard M. Kravitz

Recent neurobiological advances have been applied to the clarification and understanding of the biological bases of psychiatric illnesses. Researchers have elucidated neurochemical, neuroendocrine, and neurophysiological concomitants of affective illness as the basis for the development or the perpetuation of these disorders. Clinicians have attempted to use data from these biological models to assist in differential diagnosis and to predict likely responsiveness to various somatic treatments.

Although depression has been reported to be the most prevalent psychiatric disorder, the true prevalence of this disorder is unknown. Community surveys based upon depression symptom scales have yielded a current depression point prevalence rate of up to 20% (Boyd & Weissman, 1981; Weissman & Myers, 1978a). Using a structured interview, the Schedule for Affective Disorders and Schizophrenia (SADS), and the Research Diagnostic Criteria (RDC) (Endicott & Spitzer, 1978; Endicott & Spitzer, 1979; Spitzer et al., 1978b), Weissman and associates (Weissman & Myers, 1978b; Weissman et al., 1978) found a combined current point prevalence rate of 6.8% for major (4.3%) and minor (2.5%) depression. Lifetime prevalence rates were 20% (18% definite) for major and 9.2% (8.6% definite) for minor depression, for a combined rate of 26.7% for probable and definite depressions, and 24.7% for definite diagnoses only. Unipolar depression is twice as common in women as in men. Bipolar affective disorders (Bipolar I and Bipolar II) have a reported lifetime prevalence rate of

1.2%, with a slight female sex predominance. Further, about 15% of affective disorder patients successfully commit suicide (Avery & Winokur, 1978), making this a potentially fatal disorder. Data from the Collaborative Program on the Psychobiology of Depression have revealed interesting findings on symptoms and longitudinal course in this heterogenous group of disorders lumped under the rubic of "depression."

In view of the significance of affective illness, particularly depression, the demonstration of potential *psychobiological markers*—including trait markers of vulnerability and susceptibility to illness and state markers that may help to monitor the course of an episode as well as suggest a course of beneficial treatment alternatives—would be welcome findings. The ability of these biological correlates of illness to suggest potential differential responsivity to treatment is especially important given the likelihood of recurrence of these disorders and their eminent treatability if approached early and aggressively. Unrecognized, untreated, and poorly-treated depressions contribute heavily to the chronicity and treatment-resistance found in depressive illness; 10% to 20% of unipolar major depressives and 33% of bipolar patients have a chronic course (Clayton, 1981; Keller et al., 1982; Murphy et al., 1974; Weissman & Klerman, 1977).

In this chapter we present some of the latest findings in the psychobiological research in affective illness, particularly depressive disorders. We will specifically review the clinical applicability of these findings and their influence upon diagnostic and treatment-oriented decision-making processes.

DIAGNOSTIC ISSUES

Because depression is a heterogenous group of disorders, its diagnosis and classification remain controversial. Further confusion has come about through the unresolved relationship of clinical phenomenology, or phenomenologic subtype, to biological factors, or biological subtype. Prior to the advances brought about through psychobiological research, classificatory schemes were based solely on phenomenological features. The Feighner criteria developed by the St. Louis group (Feighner et al., 1972) preceded the development of the RDC (Spitzer, et al., 1978a) and, most recently, the Diagnostic and Statistical Manual III (DSM-III) (American Psychiatric Association, 1980). The present emphasis is on developing biological correlates of these disorders. Through additional knowledge provided by genetics and neurobiology, biological differences among depressives have been found, and attempts have been made at delineating biologically homogenous groups of depression.

These various biological classifications make the assumption that biological factors in some way reflect the underlying etiology of these illnesses. Evidence that certain depressive subtypes, particularly melancholia, are associated with alterations in central nervous system (CNS) functioning continues to accumulate.

However, it has not been established that these changes cause depression or even how these changes come about. The ancient Greeks believed that the liver removed toxic humors, including black bile, from food. Hepatic dysfunction was though to result in excessive accumulation of black bile and thereby produce severe depression or melancholia Today, affective illnesses are thought to be associated with accumulations or deficiencies of other body humors–brain neurotransmitters.

BIOGENIC AMINE HYPOTHESES OF AFFECTIVE ILLNESS

Over the past quarter-century it has been proposed that affective disorders are principally related to monoamine system dysfunction. The major focus has been on functional changes in the central noradrenergic and serotonergic systems. These theories arose from observations that antidepressants and stimulants activate brain monoamine synapses while drugs such as reserpine, which induce depression, reduce monoamine transmission (Brodie & Costa, 1962; Brodie & Shore, 1957). Although we have yet to determine the exact mechanism by which the antidepressant action of drugs is produced, the most widely held view suggests that it is mediated through effects on central catecholamines (CA), norepinephrine (NE) and dopamine (DA), and indoleamines (IA), principally serotonin (5-HT). Thus, antidepressants, including tricyclics (TCA) and monoamine oxidase inhibitors (MAOI), are thought to enhance the availability of functionally active NE at the synaptic cleft of noradrenergic neurons. Challenges to these hypotheses have arisen from studies demonstrating the efficacy of "atypical" antidepressants (such as mianserin and iprindole), which appear to act by different mechanisms (Zis & Goodwin, 1979).

Recent animal models of TCA effects suggest that they act by down-modulating CA-receptor systems, thereby decreasing receptor sensitivity, compatible with emerging evidence that TCA might work by inhibiting noradrenergic activity by producing (postsynaptic) receptor subsensitivity (Sulser, 1982; Sulser et al., 1978; Vetulani & Sulser, 1975). Similarly, MAOI may produce a relative brain NE-deficit by preferentially raising brain levels of nonhydroxylated amines, such as phenylethylamine (PEA) and tyramine. Further study of postsynaptic receptor function may provide more information about biochemical events associated with depressive illness.

Catecholamine Hypothesis

The dominant biogenic amine hypothesis, especially in the United States, has been the *catecholamine hypothesis*. Initially posited by Schildkraut (1965), and Bunney and Davis (1965), it states in its simplest terms that some if not all depressions are related to an absolute or relative brain NE deficiency at functionally important adrenergic receptor sites, while manic disorders are associated with functional excesses of CA transmission. This hypothesis has developed within a clinically oriented framework over the past two decades. In an attempt to demonstrate disturbed CA metabolism referable to the CNS, much research focused on the measurement of NE and its metabolites. One of the most intensively studied metabolites has been 3-methoxy-4-hydroxyphenylglycol (MHPG). Reports suggested that while vanillylmandelic acid (VMA) is the major NE metabolite measured in the urine (Ebert & Kopin, 1975), MHPG is the major brain NE metabolite reflecting CNS turnover (Axelrod et al., 1959; Maas & Landis, 1971; Maas et al., 1979; Maas et al., 1968; Schanberg et al., 1968). Despite reports suggesting decreased brain NE turnover rates and NE depletion in depressives, as determined by the measurement of abnormally low MHPG urinary levels, there is no general consensus regarding either the exact amount of urinary MHPG which derives from the brain or its absolute urinary content. Bipolars tend to excrete less than normals or unipolars (DeLeon-Jones et al., 1975), while many depressives excrete normal or greater than normal amounts of MHPG (Schatzberg et al., 1980; Schatzberg et al., 1981; Schildkraut et al., 1978). Relatively more endogenous than nonendogenous depressives excrete MHPG in the range of bipolars (Schildkraut et al., 1978). In human subjects, a range of only 20%–70% of urinary MHPG may originate in the CNS (Blombery et al., 1980; Maas et al., 1979; Mardh et al., 1981) and 40%–50% of plasma-free MHPG may be converted to VMA (Blombery et al., 1980). Normal subjects excrete 900–3500 mcg/24 hours of MHPG, which overlaps the "pathological range" found in depressives (Fawcett et al., 1972; Goodwin & Potter, 1979; Hollister et al., 1978; Maas et al., 1968; Schatzberg et al., 1981). MHPG has also been examined in other body fluids, including cerebrospinal fluid (CSF) and plasma, again with inconclusive results regarding clinical usefulness (DeMet & Halaris, 1979; Kopin et al., 1983). The relationships between urinary, plasma and CSF MHPG are still not completely understood.

Thus, controversy exists regarding the methodology behind these findings, their consistency and reliability, and their interpretation. MHPG may be affected by such variables as age, sex, and clinical state. MHPG levels may represent an epiphenomenon related to anxiety or activity (Ko et al., 1983; Sweeney et al., 1978), especially as anxiety and depression often coexist clinically (Fawcett & Kravitz, 1983). However, state anxiety and urinary MHPG may not co-vary significantly (Sweeney et al., 1978).

Despite considerable debate, studies of urinary MHPG support the CA hypothesis to the extent that a CA deficit plays a role in some but not all forms of depressive illness. On the other hand, an excess of brain CA is thought to account for mania. Although no data indicate that manics as a group excrete greater amounts of MHPG than normals, they do excrete significantly more during manic or normal periods than during depressive episodes (Jones et al., 1973). This has been explained by a "switch process" associated with cycling from one affective state to another (Bunney et al., 1972; Wehr et al., 1980). Further, treatment with alpha-methyl-para-tyrosine (AMPT), an inhibitor of tyrosine hydroxylase, the enzyme catalyzing the synthesis of NE and DA, lessened mania in five of seven manics and worsened depression in the three depressives, as well as decreased MHPG, VMA, and DA in all ten patients (Brodie et al., 1971).

Less studied is the relationship between DA, the other major CA, and its major CSF metabolite, homovanillic acid (HVA), in affective illness (Randrup et al., 1975). A similar too little–too much relationship in depressives and manics, respectively, is thought to exist (Randrup & Braestrup, 1977). CSF HVA measurements may have some value in differentiating depressive subtypes, but further investigation is necessary. Further, the DA presursor L-dopa may induce hypomania or mania, but not reverse depressive processes, suggesting that these two disorders may actually be separable processes rather than opposite poles of a single biochemical continuum (Goodwin et al., 1970; Murphy et al., 1971; Murphy et al., 1973).

How can we interpret data relating MHPG and treatment response to the CA hypothesis of affective disorders? Blackwell (1979) designated this potential biological marker the "*M*yth of *H*eterogenous *P*sychiatric *G*roups." Treatment studies have demonstrated that while imipramine (IMI) responders had significantly lower MHPG urinary excretion compared with normals and with amitriptyline (AMI) responders (Beckmann & Goodwin, 1975), both increases and decreases have been observed following antidepressant treatment (Beckmann & Goodwin, 1975; Fawcett et al., 1972; Maas et al., 1972). Further, MHPG levels have been found to be reduced in nonresponders (Beckmann & Goodwin, 1975; Beckmann et al., 1975). These contradictory pre- and post-antidepressant treatment MHPG data suggest these data must be cautiously interpreted.

Veith and associates (1983) found that pre-treatment urinary MHPG alone did not adequately predict the treatment response to AMI and desipramine (DMI) in unipolar depressives. MHPG response to these two drugs indicated that TCA response may be mediated through effects other than alterations of NE alone. Maas and associates (1982) examined the pre-treatment CSF 5-hydroxyindoleacetic acid (5-HIAA), MHPG, HVA, and urinary MHPG, and the response of these metabolites to IMI and AMI treatment, in 87 depressives in the National Institute of Mental Health (NIMH) Collaborative Study on the Psychobiology of Depression. On the basis of baseline amine levels and outcome of drug treatment they postulated a subtype characterized by low MHPG and/or low CSF 5-HIAA, responsive to IMI, implying either independent changes in neuronal system function or an interactive relationship between these two monoamine systems.

Indoleamine Hypothesis

While the role of CA in affective disorders was being investigated in the United States, similar studies were being undertaken with 5-hydroxytryptamine (serotonin, 5-HT) in Europe. The "indoleamine hypothesis of affective illness" states that functional brain 5-HT levels are reduced and may directly contribute to or predispose to symptoms of depression and possibly mania (Coppen, 1967). This hypothesis is based on findings that reserpine and antidepressants affect 5-HT in essentially similar ways as they affect CA and on the results of 5-HT precursor and metabolite studies (Kalin et al., 1981; Lapin & Oxenkrug, 1969; Murphy et al., 1978; Van Praag, 1981). Most studies have reported that CSF 5-HIAA, the major 5-HT metabolite, is reduced in at least a subgroup of depressives compared with controls; no study found significantly higher levels in patient groups. Asberg and associates (1976) found a bimodal distribution, suggesting a low 5-HIAA subgroup, which may be due to an over-representation of males in the low group (Murphy et al., 1978) or a bimodal distribution in the phases of 24-hour 5-HT rhythms without change in the total 24-hour turnover (Kripke, 1976). Most groups have reported low or normal baseline and probenecid-induced 5-HIAA accumulations in manics, though the probenecid-induced levels were less than in controls or unipolar depressives (Murphy et al., 1978; Zis & Goodwin, 1982). Manics as well as bipolar depressives may represent a subgroup without a 5-HT deficit, though opposing data have been presented (Coppen, 1972; Prange et al., 1974).

Treatment studies suggest that there may be a 5-HT deficient biological subtype of depression. For example, nortriptyline (NT), a putative NE-reuptake blocker, has been reported to effectively treat depressives with high baseline CSF 5-HIAA; however, both 5-HIAA and indole-3-acetic acid significantly decreased in responders and nonresponders, indicating that NT inhibits 5-HT reuptake as well (Asberg et al., 1973). Thus, although a reduced CSF 5-HIAA may reflect the hypothesized brain 5-HT deficit, the origin of the dysfunction is still not clear (e.g., synthesis and/or metabolic dysfunction).

Phenylethylamine Hypothesis
of Affective Behavior

Although CA and 5-HT continue to be central to biochemical theories of depression, other endogenous neurochemicals and neurotransmitters must also be considered to play at least a contributory role. An amine which has received much less widespread attention is PEA. The "PEA hypothesis of affective behavior," proposed by Sabelli and Mosnaim (1974), states that PEA is a neuromodulator responsible for sustaining attention and mood. PEA is formed from the dietary amino acid phenylalanine. It is pharmacologically, structurally, and metabolically related to CA and to amphetamine, and produces amphetamine-like behavioral and electrophysiological effects; for these reasons it is thought to be an endogenous amphetamine. Because it crosses the blood-brain barrier PEA is considered a neuromodulator rather than a neurotransmitter per se; its biological actions are partly mediated by CA release, thus possibly acting via modulation of brain CA synapses. Although PEA excretion is low and variable, most of it is metabolized by monoamine oxidase (MAO) type B to phenylacetic acid (PAA), which is excreted in milligram rather than microgram or nanogram amounts, and is thus more readily measured. We have found that PAA urinary excretion is markedly decreased in about 60% of depressives and increased in 44% of manics (normal range 70–175 mg./24 hours in 70% of controls) (Sabelli et al., 1983a, 1983b), and it returns to normal with the resolution of an episode of illness. Although antidepressant drugs in general increase PAA levels, no great difference in these levels has been found between untreated and ineffectively treated depressives. This excretion is not affected by sex or normal mood variation, but may be elevated in anxiety states (unpublished observations). Thus, we suspect that these changes may provide a state marker for assisting in the diagnosis and monitoring of the course and treatment of affective disorders. Further support comes from Sandler and associates' (1979) findings of lower CSF PAA levels in "primary depressive illness" as compared with controls. However, these observations relating PEA and/or PAA levels to affective states have been criticized on methodological and biochemical grounds as well as on the clinical definition of depressive syndromes. Relating PAA excretion to PAA metabolism in brain implies an assumption not empirically supported. There are no data regarding the relative proportions which brain and peripheral tissues contribute to urinary PAA. Clinically, the test is nonspecific. Depressive subtype, including unipolar and bipolar, cannot be differentiated, and low excretion has been noted in a subgroup of manics and in chronic schizophrenics (Potkin et al., 1980). There are no normative data from other psychiatric or medical disorders. We are presently studying plasma PAA in control subjects. Thus, the interpretation and understanding of these findings remain an open question.

Two-Amine Hypotheses

Single amine hypotheses appear to represent oversimplifications and do not account for the adaptive and complex function of the nervous system. Certainly neither pharmacologic studies, which include precursor loading techniques, nor monoamine metabolite measurements exclusively support one or the other biogenic amine hypothesis of depression.

The observation that CSF 5-HIAA levels remain low in unipolar and bipolar depressives even after recovery led to a hypothesis relating 5-HT and NE in depression—the "permissive hypothesis" (Mendels & Frazer, 1975; Prange et al., 1974). Thus, low 5-HT turnover interacts with alterations in CA, rendering individuals chronically chemically susceptible to depression or mania depending upon the direction of changes in CA levels. These affective swings are "permitted" by the low 5-HT, which must be present for the clinical expression of this chemical vulnerability to be manifested, and acute mood changes represent alterations in CA levels.

Shortly after Beckmann and Goodwin (1975) reported differential drug responsivity based on MHPG level (high or normal versus low), Maas (1975) defined two possible biological subtypes of depression, based on the following biochemical and pharmacological criteria.

1. Type A is characterized by
(a) low pretreatment urinary MHPG
(b) favorable clinical response to IMI or DMI, which is predicted by mood improvement following a brief trial or challenge with dextroamphetamine (Fawcett & Siomopoulos, 1971)
(c) modest increment or no change in MHPG following any of these three drugs (although decrements have also been reported [Beckmann & Goodwin, 1975])
(d) failure to respond to AMI
2. Type B is characterized by
(a) normal or high urinary MHPG
(b) a favorable response to AMI
(c) Lack of favorable mood response following dextroamphetamine challenge or treatment with IMI or DMI
(d) MHPG decrement following any of these three latter drugs.

Maas specified that Type A depressions were related to altered central noradrenergic systems, while Type B probably instead reflected a disturbance in 5-HT system function. He was careful to point out only that "serotonin *appears* to be a worthwhile candidate for investigation," and never definitively stated that Type B was a serotonin-depletion depression. Further, dopaminergic mechanisms may be involved in mania, but this disorder was not well explained by this model.

Schildkraut and associates (1981) have modified the CA hypothesis, proposing at least three subtypes based on MHPG excretion (less than 1950 mcg/24 hr, 1950–2500 mcg/24hr; greater than 2500 mcg/24 hr). Each subgroup may be differentially responsive to TCA therapy (Schatzberg et al., 1981). Interaction with 5-HT and acetylcholine (ACh) may occur in the intermediate and high MHPG subgroups, respectively. Thus, urinary MHPG may be useful, though not adequate by itself, for subtyping depressions and assessing biochemical specificity of drug action, even if the majority of this MHPG is of peripheral origin. It may not be the measure of choice to reflect the imbalance in monoamine transmission (Koslow et al., 1983).

Sabelli and associates (1983c) described an alternative to Maas' approach: Types 1 and II depressive subtypes. Type 1 may be associated with depletion in various monoamine systems, including NE, 5-HT, and PEA, and responsiveness to IMI-like antidepressants. On the other hand, Type II may involve a PEA deficit, reflected in reduced urinary PAA in AMI-responders (Sabelli et al., unpublished data) without concomitant NE or 5-HT depletion. Type II depressives appear responsive to both AMI- and NT-like antidepressants.

Major impediments encountered in attempting to interpret drug response and amine metabolite correlation studies are the differing criteria for defining depression and the lack of report of all relevant monoamines in each patient study. In a large multicenter study, investigators from the Collaborative Program on the Psychobiology of Depression—Biological Studies (Koslow et al., 1983) collected baseline CSF 5-HIAA, HVA and MHPG, and urinary NE, epinephrine, VMA, normetanephrine, metanephrine, and MHPG. The data obtained suggested an abnormality and/or imbalance of neuroamine transmission in depressives compared with healthy controls. The relationship of these various amines and their metabolites to depressive subtypes, clinical states, symptomatology, and behavior requires elaboration. The relative importance of the various monoamines, and their relevant interactions, are frequently speculated upon but are still open to investigation. The possibility that monoamine levels reflect an epiphenomenon related to patient variables such as activity, anxiety, gender, body build, and nutritional status, as well as factors affecting the amine system(s) independently (such as receptor changes) rather than depression per se must still be considered. Despite theoretical disagreements about monoamines and affective illness, psychiatrists have observed that patients who do not respond to one type of TCA (e.g., 5-HT reuptake blockers such as AMI) may respond to another type (e.g., DMI, a NE reuptake blocker). However, no controlled crossover study demonstrating this has been published. This leads to the question of whether differential drug response constitutes more than inferential support for any underlying mechanism at the level of neuronal synapses in the brain. It is important to distinguish between neuronal systems that are directly involved in producing or maintaining and affecting a disease process and those that are indirectly involved, the result of a disease process. Changes in metabolic by-products of monoamines may be epiphenomena. Interestingly, although the biochemical hypotheses are derived from observations of the effects of various drugs on biochemical variables as well as therapeutic effects, the clinical observations of treatment response continue to make up a major source of evidence supporting these various biochemical hypotheses. A decade ago Baldessarini (1975) critically evaluated the biogenic amine hypotheses of affective disorders.

Today, we have increased our data base, but still the riddle of "what makes that so" is unanswered.

NEUROENDOCRINE HYPOTHESES

Amid the turmoil of contradictory findings, criticism, and controversy regarding monoamine system dysfunction, changes in limbic system and hypothalamic function that may imply altered CA and/or 5-HT function have been virtually unchallenged as the primary mechanisms of biochemical changes associated with affective illness. Further, affective symptoms, including depressed mood, vegetative symptoms, autonomic symptoms, and diurnal variation (circadian rhythm), suggest hypothalamic dysfunction. Complex regulatory mechanisms and interactions involve neurotransmitter systems as well as hypothalamic and pituitary-releasing and inhibitory factors. Thus, the study of neuroendocrine function may be another strategy for evaluating affective illnesses as well as the biogenic amine hypotheses (Checkley, 1980).

Limbic System–Hypothalamic–Pituitary–
Adrenal Axis (LHPA)

Early studies showing hyperactivity of the pituitary–adrenal axis manifested by elevations of cortisol secretion rates, corticosteroid metabolic breakdown products, and urine-free cortisol as well as blood and CSF cortisol in some severely depressed patients, supported a concept of adrenal activation associated with some forms of depressive illness (Fawcett & Bunney, 1967; Rubin & Mandell, 1966). Studies of altered circadian pituitary function revealed a disturbed circadian control of HPA function in many depressives (Krieger et al., 1971; Sachar et al., 1973). That this is not the consequence of "ego defense breakdown" was demonstrated by Carroll (1976).

Following the midnight oral administration of 2 mg. of dexamethasone (dexamethasone suppression test, DST), a potent artificial glucocorticoid that usually induces absolute suppression of HPA activity by blocking release of adrenocorticotropic hormone (ACTH), plasma cortisol levels were drawn at 8:30 a.m. and 4:30 p.m. (8 ½ and 16 ½ hours later). Persistent elevation of plasma cortisol in the depressed patients as compared with the schizophrenics indicated that the HPA activation and nonsuppression was related to the depressive illness itself. This "disinhibition" of the normal CNS regulatory influences within the LHPA has been linked with the process of the primary depressive illness, or "endogenous" (melancholic) features rather than the depressed mood per se (Carroll, 1982; Carroll et al., 1981; Feinberg & Carroll, 1982). The origin of this cortisol dysregulation is thought to be suprahypophyseal (i.e., in the limbic system), resulting in excessive ACTH release, rather than adrenal hyperactivity. Thus, the usual effect of dexamethasone is mediated by feedback inhibition of the system that is controlled by the hypothalamus as well as by functional connections with the limbic system. Failure to suppress suggests an abnormal state of activation in the LHPA. Further, no data indicate that the disinhibition is an etiological factor in the development of depressive disorders despite its temporal association. The neural basis for this disinhibition remains uncertain. However, the alterations in the neurochemical links between the limbic system of the brain and the anterior pituitary may involve disturbances in central monoamine systems, producing an override of both circadian and feedback systems. Amsterdam and associates (1983) performed an ACTH stimulation test as well as the oral DST in 16 female patients with major depressive disorder, endogenous subtype, and 11 age- and sex-matched controls, and found a greater cortisol release and earlier peak response after ACTH infusion as well as a lack of association between cortisol response and the DST result. They suggested that the cortisol hypersecretion in their depressives could have resulted from adrenocortical hyper-responsiveness.

This HPA dysfunction in response to dexamethasone suppression is more subtle than that associated with Cushing's disease. True Cushing's patients do not suppress even at higher dexamethasone doses. In response to the now-established standard 1 mg. (Carroll, 1982; Carroll et al., 1981) oral dose of dexamethasone administered at 11:00 p.m. (between 11:00 p.m. and midnight, to account for circadian periodicity of cortisol secretion), a subgroup of depressives demonstrated abnormal "early escape" from suppression. Although earlier studies reported 8:00 a.m., 4:00 p.m., and 11:00 p.m. post-dexamethasone cortisol levels, the DST has been modified for outpatient use, and requires only a 4:00 p.m. blood sample. Although this results in a lower sensitivity for the test, it is still reported as a useful outpatient procedure. An elevated cortisol at any time within 24 hours after dexamethasone administration (nonsuppression) is a positive test. The cut-off value for cortisol may vary, depending upon the laboratory and method used, but generally is considered to be 4 mcg % by radioimmunoassay and 5 mcg % by competitive protein binding techniques.

Although many claims have been made for the use and value of the DST, its sensitivity is only about 50%, specificity is about 95%, and the predictive value of a positive test is about 90%. This latter value, however, is deceptive, and it depends upon the prevalence rate of melancholia, or endogenous depression, in the population sample studied. Evidence to date points to its potential value for serial testing, both for monitoring recovery from affective illness if the initial test was positive (a state-dependent marker) as well for predicting relapse (conversion to nonsuppression). In a thoughtful critical review of the available data, Insel and Goodwin (1983) concluded that a positive test neither assists in the differential diagnosis among depressions or between depression and other diagnostic categories, nor implies treatment-responsive or genetic subgroups of depression. Thus, although the DST is in widespread clinical use, we still do not know enough about its interpretation to recommend its routine use in the clinical diagnosis and management of depression (Hirschfield et al., 1983).

Limbic System-Hypothalamic-Pituitary-Thyroid Axis (LHPT)

Investigation of the relationship between depression and the HPT axis has arisen through observations of the effects of thyroid dysfunction on mood states. Brain monoamines may play a role in the thyroid stimulating hormone (TSH) response to thyroid releasing hormone (TRH): NE stimulates TRH cells and subsequent hypothalamic TRH release; 5-HT has mainly an inhibitory role; and DA demonstrates some stimulating effect, though is inactive when its conversion to NE is blocked (Martin et al., 1977). Further, TSH has a circadian rhythm, with a nocturnal rise, and is modulated by TRH, which facilitates release, and by thyroid hormones, which give feedback inhibition of release. Beyond this level, our understanding of the interactions between monoamine neurotransmitters, receptors, and the thyroid and its hormones is speculative and incomplete (Whybrow and Prange, 1981).

Working independently, Prange et al. (1972) and Kastin et al. (1972) demonstrated a diminished (blunted) pituitary TSH response to an intravenous infusion of TRH (protirelin) in patients with normal baseline thyroid hormone levels, as well as an occasional brief antidepressant effect. Ten years later, a review of 47 studies involving 963 patients revealed that all but 5 studies involving 36 patients reported findings consistent with the initial results (Loosen & Prange, 1982). Depending upon the criterion value chosen, blunted responses have been reported in 25%–50% of patients with major depression (more so in unipolars than bipolars), in contrast to few in nondepressives, minor depressives, schizophrenics, or normal volunteers (Baldessarini, 1983; Targum, 1983). However, the mechanism, as well as the functional significance of this blunted response, is still incompletely understood, and the interpretation of the data obtained is uncertain. While it may be a state and/or trait marker, it does not seem to be related to the cause of depression. It may be useful in unmasking subclinical hypo- and hyperthyroidism, long recognized as causes of affective and behavioral disorders (Whybrow & Prange, 1981), although in patients with psychiatric disorders and a blunted TSH response to TRH there has been no clinical evidence for pituitary or thyroid disease, and most patients have normal baseline thyroid function (Loosen & Prange, 1982).

The sequential use of DST and TRH tests has been studied. The basis for each abnormality seems to be different, and only 11%–30% of depressions manifest both abnormalities (Extein et al., 1981; Loosen et al., 1978; Targum et al., 1982). Importantly, the order of the two tests matters; the glucocorticoid dexamethasone may cause TSH blunting, and therefore the TRH stimulation test should be performed first (Targum et al., 1982).

Growth Hormone and Affective Illness

Pituitary growth hormone (GH) is secreted episodically in response to stress (via limbic system connections); metabolic and neural factors (via hypothalamic and extrahypothalamic limbic system connections); and pharmacologic stimulation. Its maximal daily surge in blood occurs at 24-hour intervals within the first 2 hours after sleep onset, coinciding with the first appearance of slow-wave sleep (delta sleep, stages 3 and 4) (Boyar, 1978). Its activity may be regulated by various neurotransmitter systems; release may be stimulated by alpha-adrenergic, dopaminergic, and serotonergic agonists, and beta-adrenergic antagonists (Blackard & Heidingsfelder, 1968). Thus, study of GH secretion has been associated with models directed toward understanding the role of CNS aminergic receptors in the amine hypotheses of depressive disorders.

Abnormal (diminished) GH secretion in response to various pharmacologic challenges have been reported in depressive disorders. These studies have focused on GH response to insulin-induced hypoglycemia, to noradrenergic and dopaminergic agonists (i.e., amphetamine, L-dopa, clonidine, desipramine, apomorphine), to TRH administration, and to altered sleep-induced release. Although Gold and associates (1976) have reported unipolar–bipolar differences, no consistent abnormalities have been found. Most of these studies have been criticized for the lack of adequate control for age, sex and menopausal status (high estrogen may elevate basal GH concentration), body weight (should not deviate more than 20% of ideal body weight) and, in the case of insulin-induced hypoglycemia, a lack of an established minimum decrement from baseline plasma glucose levels (should fall at least 50%). Further, baseline GH should be less than or equal to 5ng/ml, and preferably less than 3ng/ml. Preliminary data from the Collaborative Program on the Psychobiology of Depression could not support the hypothesis of altered hypothalamic-pituitary-growth hormone system function in depression (Koslow et al., 1982). Although unipolar depressives had significantly greater resistance to insulin-induced hypoglycemia, the mean peak GH concentrations were not significantly different between unipolars, bipolars and normal controls, although bipolars had greater range and variability in this peak response. Thus, explanation and interpretation of abnormal results await definition of a true abnormal result from rigorously defined criteria established among normal controls. The general usefulness of challenge tests and GH function in affective illness is presently limited.

THE STIMULANT CHALLENGE TEST

The observation that dextroamphetamine, a potent NE uptake blocker, may produce transient mood elevation in depressives (especially those with low MHPG who may later respond to TCA) lends further support to both the biogenic amine hypothesis and to the possibility that MHPG may be a relevant biochemical marker in depression. Independent of the biochemical theories, the possibility still exists that a provocative or challenge test predictive of response to treatment may be found. Despite the widespread use of antidepressant drugs, prediction of individual therapeutic response to specific agents is still an important unsolved problem.

Dextroamphetamine and its congeners—such as methylphenidate (Ritalin)— are known to exert rapid mood effects despite limited efficacy as true antidepressants, in contrast to the delayed and gradual yet lasting effect of antidepressants. However, there is a wide range of individual differences in behavioral response to stimulants, mediated primarily by NE. These facts led to the hypothesis that a test dose of dextroamphetamine might predict a therapeutic response to TCA.

Fawcett and Siomopoulos (1971) initially reported that dextroamphetamine was a useful research drug for studying biochemical-behavioral interactions. Subsequent reports by Fawcett and associates (Fawcett & Siomopoulos, 1971; Fawcett et al., 1972; Fawcett et al., 1983b; Maas et al., 1972; Sabelli et al., 1983c) and others (Van Kammen & Murphy, 1975; 1978; 1979) suggested that patients can be differentiated on the basis of behavioral responses to dextroamphetamine or methylphenidate. The primary value of this safe, simple, rapid, and noninvasive procedure may be to distinguish biochemically different depressive subtypes and to predict specific TCA response in individual patients.

Although there is a continuum of observable responses, responders and nonresponders can be separated on the basis of mood ratings. In our clinical experience, the delayed and overall effects of oral doses of dextroamphetamine or methylphenidate over a period of at least two days is more indicative of future TCA treatment response than short-lasting mood changes. It is crucial to distinguish euphoriant from antidepressant responses; the former tend to be of shorter onset and duration (Checkley, 1978). We administer either drug for 1–3 days, using the patient's subjective mood response to select TCA treatment (we do not have adequate data regarding prediction of MAOI response). We have precipitated manic episodes with this challenge test in bipolar depressives, but no psychotic episodes in our affective disorder patients. Although we have found little clinical difference between the two stimulants, some patients preferentially respond to one or the other; with nonresponsive patients we sequentially employ the two, as pharmacological studies suggest potential important differences (Brown et al., 1978). A positive response consists of mood elevation as well as manic euphoria, whereas increased energy or motor activity alone are not. Negative responses include dysphoric anxiety or agitation.

As reported earlier, in a naturalistic nondouble-blind study, Sabelli and associates (1983c) noted that patients responding favorably to methylphenidate responded to IMI or DMI, but not to NT or AMI, while methylphenidate-negative patients responsive to AMI maintained this response despite substitution with NT (adequate plasma levels attained with all TCA). Although this suggests that NT may be more similar to AMI in its pharmacological and biochemical activity profile, one must remember that antidepressant efficacy may occur through another mechanism, such as alteration in receptor sensitivities. Another potential criticism of this model is the fact that all neurotransmitter systems, including NE, 5-HT, DA, PEA, ACh, may be important in the brain, and therefore it may be presumptuous to attribute behavioral effects to the action of TCA and stimulants on any one system. Further, subjective reports and behavioral observations may be discrepant, and the interpretation of partial responses is currently another unsolved enigma. We are currently studying the correlation between biological and behavioral responses to stimulants, using PAA excretion and stimulant-induced change in excretion, in order to discern a biochemical basis for the mood-elevating effect of the stimulants, as well as a pleasure scale that will determine whether concomitant changes occur in hedonic capacity (Fawcett et al., 1983a).

Others have attempted to correlate the response to stimulants with neuroendocrinological changes in order to clarify neurochemical alterations in depressive disorders (Risch et al., 1981; Siever et al., 1982). Contrary to the hypothesis that DST nonsuppression indicates a central noradrenergic deficiency state (Carroll et al., 1981), significant negative correlations have been found between DST and methylphenidate responsiveness (dexamethasone suppressors had positive mood change; nonsuppressors had a negative stimulant challenge response) (Brown and Brawley, 1983; Sternbach et al., 1981). However, 16 of 17 methylphenidate responders had a good response to IMI while 23 of 24 nonresponders to methylphenidate responded well to AMI, thus indicating future antidepressant responsiveness, as predicted by Fawcett and associates (Fawcett & Siomopoulos, 1971; Fawcett et al., 1972; Fawcett et al., 1983b; Maas et al., 1972; Sabelli et al., 1983c). Ettigi and associates (1983) administered 30 mg. of dextroamphetamine nonblinded to unipolar depressives and found that 10 of 13 DMI responders and 3 of 5 DMI nonresponders had a positive behavioral response; this difference was not statistically significant. Of 11 patients with an abnormal DST, 10 responded to DMI. Only 7 of the 13 DMI responders demonstrated both DST nonsuppression and positive amphetamine challenge, indicating that an NE deficiency state may be the underlying abnormality in a subgroup of unipolar depressives.

Last is the issue of state versus trait. We have noted a number of patients who respond positively to a stimulant and IMI-like TCA during one depressive episode and switch responsiveness (i.e., negative stimulant response and positive AMI response) during a subsequent episode, as well as alternating pharmacological responsiveness over the course of recurrent depressions. These intraindividual changes require further investigation and elucidation.

Thus, the stimulant challenge test may be a useful clinical test for individual patients for the prediction of treatment response. In addition, pharmacological challenge tests are coming into more widespread use as research tools for distinguishing biochemically heterogenous affective disorders. State versus trait issues also require further investigation. Available studies suggest the need for replication with double-blind stimulant administration and subsequent TCA treatment as well as standardized clinical criteria for defining response and objective rating instruments for measuring this response. Correlations with other biochemical and neuroendocrinological measures are also desirable.

LITHIUM TRANSPORT

The clinical introduction of lithium produced evidence of both its antimanic and antidepressant effects acutely, as well as its prophylactic effects in these disorders, particularly in bipolar affective disorders. Recent studies of lithium effects on membrane electrolyte transport suggest that further information concerning their shifts across neuronal membranes may be important to our understanding of biochemical changes underlying these disorders. Observations to date have not generated useful hypotheses integrating these electrolyte shifts with pre- or post-synaptic functional changes. However, it has been demonstrated that while red blood cell (RBC)/plasma lithium concentration, or lithium ratio, is relatively constant over time within individuals, there is substantial interindividual variability in this ratio, as determined by lithium efflux. In 25% of manic-depressives—but not in controls, schizophrenics, or unipolar depressives— there was a marked reduction in the countertransport mechanism mediated by lithium–sodium exchange, resulting in markedly increased lithium ratios, both in vivo and in vitro (Ostrow et al., 1978). This pre-lithium treatment counterflow may be predictive of the in vivo lithium ratio, and increased lithium ratios may predict a clinical response to lithium. This defect is an intrinsic property of the RBC membrane, and interindividual variability of this lithium ratio is determined by variability in the counterflow mechanism as well as by race and blood pressure. In vivo and in vitro studies in control populations (Dorus et al., 1975; 1979), as well as study of Bipolar I patients and their families, have demonstrated that genetic polymorphism (Dorus et al., 1983) contributes to these interindividual differences as well, with a significantly higher ratio in affectively ill first degree relatives of manic-depressive probands independent of whether the ill relative had unipolar or bipolar illness. Genetic polymorphism at this major gene locus may be the basis for the control of lithium ratio as well as vulnerability to affective illness (Dorus, 1983).

Thus, although further investigation is required, there is early indication for the potential utility of the lithium ratio as a trait marker for susceptible populations of affective illness and as a predictor of lithium responsiveness (Ostrow et al., 1982).

BRAIN IMAGING

In recent years we have advanced beyond computerized axial tomography, which discerns structure alone; we can now directly visualize regional brain activity, i.e., brain function. These latest noninvasive radiologic procedures, which involve less radiation exposure, are positron emission tomography (PET scan) and nuclear magnetic resonance (NMR) (Brownell et al., 1982). Although information about their basic principles is accumulating, much less is known about the applicability of these techniques to the study of affective illness (Bunney et al., 1983). Neuroreceptor site concentration flow can be studied with PET; this may be a method for observing and understanding drug activity at receptor sites in the brain. We expect to hear more about these exciting new techniques and their potential clinical and research applications in the future.

CONCLUSIONS

The biological basis for affective illness has generated a vast amount of literature with a wide variety of approaches, making any attempt to review and evaluate it an overwhelming task. We have attempted to review the relevant developments in this area in order to provide an understanding of the current state of research in the field. Research into the neurochemistry and neurophysiology of affective illness has yet to produce proof of any particular biological hypothesis. The most striking feature of all the data relating to the various biogenic amine hypotheses is the inconsistency, including heterogeneity of patients and clinical syndromes, variability of study conditions, lack of sensitivity and specificity of metabolic measurements and assays, and multiple actions and effects of pharmacologic agents on neurotransmitter systems. Further, acute versus chronic effects of drugs on receptors need to be considered. We must remember that these are dynamic, not static systems. Phenomenological and syndromal differences in affective syndromes and characteristics of responses to somatic treatments must be related to highly specific, time-related and often contradictory findings at different locations in the nervous system. In order to develop a true biobehavioral understanding of psychobiological processes, the psychological processes cannot be separated from their role in biological processes. All of these mechanisms need to be integrated.

With the possible exception of the delineation of specific drug-responsive depressive subtypes (e.g., Type A versus B, or Type I versus II depressions) and potential biochemical, pharmacologic, or neurophysiologic predictors (sleep EEG, DST, lithium transport, stimulant challenge) of drug responsiveness, these studies have not led to any treatment advances. Independent of the biochemical theories, the possibility still exists that laboratory or provocative test predictors of treatment response may be found. The monoamines NE and 5-HT are still of central importance, whether individually or in balance, in our attempts to understand these disorders and to develop treatments, yet other neuroregulators need to be considered, such as the endorphins and other neuropeptides (Hokfelt et al., 1980).

Techniques to study the complex actions and interactions of these neurotransmitters have been developed. Neuroendocrine techniques have been thought to offer a "window on the brain," sleep EEG provides a neurophysiologic approach, and neuroradiologic advances are beginning to offer a view of function as well as structure. We look forward to the further development of these exciting new techniques, and hope that they will offer us the means by which we can further understand the function of the brain in the origin of affective illness as well as provide more general information regarding the psychobiology of emotions.

Acknowledgements

Our grateful thanks to Ms. Nancy Bradley for typing this manuscript.

REFERENCES

American Psychiatric Association. (1980). *Diagnostic and statistical manual of mental disorders* (3rd ed.). Washington, DC: American Psychiatric Association.

Amsterdam, J. D., Winokur, A., Abelman, E., Lucki, I., & Rickels, K. (1983). Cosyntropin (ACTH$_{\alpha1-24}$) stimulation test in depressed patients and healthy subjects. *American Journal of Psychiatry, 140,* 907–909.

Asberg, M., Bertilsson, L., Tuck, D., Cronholm, B., & Sjoqvist, F. (1973). Indoleamine metabolites in the cerebrospinal fluid of depressed patients before and during treatment with nortriptyline. *Clinical Pharmacology and Therapeutics, 14,* 277–286.

Asberg, M., Thoren, P., Traskman, L., Bertilsson, L., & Ringberger, V. (1976). "Serotonin depression"—A biochemical subgroup within the affective disorders? *Science, 191,* 478–480.

Avery, D., & Winokur, G. (1978). Suicide, attempted suicide, and relapse rates in depression: Occurrence after ECT and antidepressant therapy. *Archives of General Psychiatry, 35,* 749–753.

Axelrod, J., Kopin, I. J., & Mann, J. D. (1959). 3-Methoxy-4-hydroxyphenylglycol sulfate: A new metabolite of epinephrine and norepinephrine. *Biochemica et Biophysica Acta, 36,* 576–577.

Baldessarini, R. J. (1975). The basis for amine hypotheses in affective disorders: A critical evaluation. *Archives of General Psychiatry, 32,* 1087–1093.

Baldessarini, R. J. (1983). *Biomedical aspects of depression and its treatment.* Washington, D.C.: American Psychiatric Press, Inc.

Beckmann, H., & Goodwin, F. K. (1975). Antidepressant response to tricyclics and urinary MHPG in unipolar patients: Clinical response to imipramine or amitriptyline. *Archives of General Psychiatry, 32,* 17–21.

Beckmann, H., St. Laurent, J., & Goodwin, F. K. (1975). The effect of lithium on urinary MHPG in unipolar and bipolar depressed patients. *Psychopharmacologia, 42,* 277–282.

Blackard, W. G., & Heidingsfelder, S. A. (1968). Adrenergic receptor control mechanism for growth hormone secretion. *Journal of Clinical Investigation, 47,* 1407–1414.

Blackwell, B. (1979). Current psychiatric research: MHPG in depression. *Psychiatric Opinion, 16,* 2, 47.

Blombery, P. A., Kopin, I. J., Gordon, E. K., Markey, S. P., & Ebert, M. H. (1980). Conversion of MHPG to vanillylmandelic acid. *Archives of General Psychiatry, 37,* 1095–1098.

Boyar, R. (1978). Sleep-related endocrine rhythms. In S. Reichlin, R. Baldessarini, & J. Martin (Eds.), *The hypothalamus* (pp. 373–386). New York: Raven Press.

Boyd, J. H., & Weissman, M. M. (1981). Epidemiology of affective disorders: A reexamination and future directions. *Archives of General Psychiatry, 38,* 1039–1046.

Brodie, B. B., & Costa, E. (1962). Some current views on brain monoamines. *Psychopharmacology Service Center Bulletin, 2,* 1–25.

Brodie, B. B., & Shore, P. A. (1957). A concept for a role of serotonin and norepinephrine as chemical mediators in the brain. *Annals of the New York Academy of Sciences, 66,* 631–642.

Brodie, H. K. H., Murphy, D. L., Goodwin, F. K., & Bunney, W. E. (1971). Catecholamines and mania: The effect of alpha-methyl-para-tyrosine on manic behavior and catecholamine metabolism. *Clinical Pharmacology and Therapeutics, 12,* 218–224.

Brown, P., & Brawley, P. (1983). Dexamethasone suppression test and mood response to methylphenidate in primary depression. *American Journal of Psychiatry, 140,* 990–993.

Brown, W. A., Corriveau, D. P., & Ebert, M. H. (1978). Acute psychologic and neuroendocrine effects of dextroamphetamine and methylphenidate. *Psychopharmacology, 58,* 189–199.

Brownell, G. L., Budinger, T. F., Lauterbaur, P. C., & McGee, P. L. (1982). Positron tomography and nuclear magnetic resonance imaging. *Science, 215,* 619–626.

Bunney, W. E., & David, J. M. (1965). Norepinephrine in depressive reactions: A review. *Archives of General Psychiatry, 13,* 483–494.

Bunney, W. E., Garland, B., & Buchsbaum, M. S. (1983). Advances in the use of visual imaging: Techniques in mental illness. *Psychiatric Annals, 13,* 420–426.

Bunney, W. E., Goodwin, F. K., Murphy, D. L., House, K. M., & Gordon, E. K. (1972). The "switch process" in manic-depressive illness. II. Relationship to catecholamines, REM sleep, and drugs. *Archives of General Psychiatry, 27,* 304–309.

Carroll, B. J. (1976). Limbic system-adrenal cortex regulation in depression and schizophrenia. *Psychosomatic Medicine, 38,* 106–121.

Carroll, B. J. (1982). The dexamethasone suppression test for melancholia. *British Journal of Psychiatry, 140,* 292–304.

Carroll, B. J., Feinberg, M., Greden, J. F., Tarika, J., Albala, A. A., Haskett, R. F., James, N. McI., Kronfol, Z., Lohr, N., Steiner, M., deVigne, J. P., & Young, E. (1981). A specific laboratory test for the diagnosis of melancholia: Standardization, validation, and clinical utility. *Archives of General Psychiatry, 38,* 15–22.

Checkley, S. A. (1978). A new distinction between the euphoric and the antidepressant effects of methylamphetamine. *British Journal of Psychiatry, 133,* 416–423.

Checkley, S. A. (1980). Neuroendocrine tests of monoamine function in man: A review of basic theory and its application to the study of depressive illness. *Psychological Medicine, 10,* 35–53.

Clayton, P. J. (1981). The epidemiology of bipolar affective disorder. *Comprehensive Psychiatry, 22,* 31–43.

Coppen, A. J. (1967). The biochemistry of affective disorders. *British Journal of Psychiatry, 113,* 1237–1264.

Coppen, A., Prange, A. J., Whybrow, P. C., & Noguera, R. (1972). Abnormalities of indoleamines in affective disorders. *Archives of General Psychiatry, 26,* 474–478.

DeLeon-Jones, F., Maas, J. W., Dekirmenjian, H., & Sanchez, J. (1975). Diagnostic subtypes of affective disorders and their urinary excretion of catecholamine metabolites. *American Journal of Psychiatry, 132,* 1141–1148.

DeMet, E. M., & Halaris, A. E. (1979). Origin and distribution of 3-methoxy-4-hydroxyphenylglycol in body fluids. *Biochemical Pharmacology, 28,* 3043–3050.

Dorus, E., Cox, N. J., Gibbons, R. D., Shaughnessy, R., Pandey, G. N. & Cloninger, C. R. (1983). Lithium ion transport and affective disorders within families of bipolar patients: Identification of a major gene locus. *Archives of General Psychiatry, 40,* 545–552.

Dorus, E., Pandey, G. N., & Davis, J. M. (1975). Genetic determinant of lithium ion distribution: An in vitro and in vivo monozygotic–dizygotic twin study. *Archives of General Psychiatry, 32,* 1097–1102.

Dorus, E., Pandey, G. N., Shaugnessy, R., Gaviria, M., Val, E., Ericksen, S., & Davis, J. M. (1979). Lithium transport across red cell membrane: A cell membrane abnormality in manic-depressive illness. *Science, 205,* 932–934.

Ebert, M. H., & Kopin, I. J. (1975). Differential labelling of origins of urinary catecholamine metabolites by dopamine-C[14]. *Transactions of the Association of American Physicians, 88,* 256–264.

Endicott, J., & Spitzer, R. L. (1978). A diagnostic interview: The Schedule for Affective Disorders and Schizophrenia. *Archives of General Psychiatry, 35,* 837–844.

Endicott, J., & Spitzer, R. L. (1979). Use of the Research Diagnostic Criteria and the Schedule for Affective Disorders and Schizophrenia to study affective disorders. *American Journal of Psychiatry, 136,* 52–56.

Ettigi, P. G., Hayes, P. E., Narasimhachari, N., Hamer, R. M., Goldberg, S., & Secord,

G. J. (1983). D-amphetamine response and dexamethasone suppression test as predictors of treatment outcome in unipolar depression. *Biological Psychiatry, 18,* 499–504.

Extein, I., Pottash, A. L. C., & Gold, M. S. (1981). Relationship of TRH test and dexamethasone suppression test abnormalities in unipolar depression. *Psychiatry Research, 4,* 49–53.

Fawcett, J., & Bunney, W. E. (1967). Pituitary adrenal function and depression: An outline for research. *Archives of General Psychiatry, 16,* 517–535.

Fawcett, J., Clark, D. C., Scheftner, W. A., & Gibbons, R. D. (1983a). Assessing anhedonia in psychiatric patients: The Pleasure Scale. *Archives of General Psychiatry, 40,* 79–84.

Fawcett, J., & Kravitz, H. M. (1983). Anxiety syndromes and their relationship to depressive illness. *Journal of Clinical Psychiatry, 44*(8, Sec. 2), 8–11.

Fawcett, J., Maas, J., & Dekirmenjian, H. (1972). Depression and MHPG excretion: Response to dextroamphetamine and tricyclic antidepressants. *Archives of General Psychiatry, 26,* 246–251.

Fawcett, J., Sabelli, H., Gusovsky, F., Epstein, P., Javaid, J., & Jeffriess, H. (1983b). Phenylethylaminic mechanisms in maprotiline antidepressant effect. *Federation Proceedings, 42,* 1164.

Fawcett, J., & Siomopoulos, V. (1971). Dextroamphetamine response as a possible predictor of improvement with tricyclic therapy in depression. *Archives of General Psychiatry, 25,* 247–255.

Feighner, J., Robins, E., Guze, S. B., Woodruff, R. A., Winokur, G., & Munoz, R. (1972). Diagnostic criteria for use in psychiatric research. *Archives of General Psychiatry, 26,* 57–63.

Feinberg, M., & Carroll, B. J. (1982). Separation of subtypes of depression using discriminant analysis. I. Separation of unipolar endogenous depression from nonendogenous depression. *British Journal of Psychiatry, 140,* 384–391.

Gold, P. W., Goodwin, F. K., Wehr, T., Rebar, R., & Sack, R. (1976). Growth-hormone and prolactin response to levodopa in affective illness. *Lancet, 2,* 1038–1309.

Goodwin, F. K., Murphy, D. L., Brodie, H. K. H., & Bunney, W. E. (1970). L-dopa, catecholamines, and behavior: A clinical and biochemical study in depressed patients. *Biological Psychiatry, 2,* 341–366.

Goodwin, F. K., & Potter, W. Z. (1979). Norepinephrine metabolite studies in affective illness. In E. Usdin, I. J. Kopin, & J. Barchas (Eds.), *Catecholamines: Basic and clinical frontiers: Vol. 2. Proceedings of the fourth international catecholamine symposium* (pp. 1863–1865). New York: Pergamon Press.

Hirschfeld, R. M. A., Koslow, S. H., & Kupfer, D. J. (1983). The clinical utility of the dexamethasone suppression test in psychiatry: Summary of the National Institute of Mental Health workshop. *Journal of the American Medical Association, 250,* 2172–2174.

Hokfelt, T., Johansson, O., Ljungdahl, A., Lundberg, J. M., & Schultzberg, M. (1980). Peptidergic neurones, *Nature, 284,* 515–521.

Hollister, L. E., Davis, K. L., Overall, L. E., & Anderson, T. (1978). Evaluation of MHPG in normal subjects. *Archives of General Psychiatry, 35,* 1410–1415.

Insel, T. R., & Goodwin, F. K. (1983). The dexamethasone suppression test: Promises and problems of diagnostic laboratory tests in psychiatry. *Hospital and Community Psychiatry, 34,* 1131–1138.

Jones, F. D., Maas, J. W., Dekirmenjian, H., & Fawcett, J. A. (1973). Urinary catecholamine metabolites during behavioral changes in a patient with manic-depressive cycles. *Science, 179,* 300–302.

Kalin, N. H., Risch, S. C., & Murphy, D. L. (1981). Involvement of the central serotonergic system in affective illness. *Journal of Clinical Psychopharmacology, 1,* 232–237.

Kastin, A. J., Ehrensing, R. H., Schalch, D. S., & Anderson, M. S. (1972). Improvement in mental depression with decreased thyrotropin response after administration of thyrotropin-releasing hormone. *Lancet, 2,* 740–742.

Keller, M. B., Klerman, G. L., Lavori, P. W., Fawcett, J. A., Coryell, W., & Endicott, J. (1982). Treatment received by depressed patients. *Journal of the American Medical Association, 248,* 1848–1855.

Ko, G. N., Elsworth, J. D. Roth, R. H., Rifkin, B. G., Leigh, H., & Redmond, D. E. (1983). Panic-induced elevation of plasma MHPG levels in phobic-anxious patients: Effects of clonidine and imipramine. *Archives of General Psychiatry, 40,* 425–430.

Kopin, I. J., Gordon, E. K., Jimerson, D. C., & Polinsky, R. J. (1983). Relation between plasma and cerebrospinal fluid levels of 3-methoxy-4-hydroxyphenylglycol. *Science, 219,* 73–75.

Koslow, S. H., Maas, J. W., Bowden, C. L., Davis, J. M., Hanin, I., & Javaid, J. (1983). CSF and urinary biogenic amines and metabolites in depression and mania: A controlled, univariate analysis. *Archives of General Psychiatry, 40,* 999–1010.

Koslow, S. H., Stokes, P. E., Mendels, J., Ramsey, A., & Casper, R. (1982). Insulin tolerance test: Human growth hormone response and insulin resistance in primary unipolar depressed, bipolar depressed and control subjects. *Psychological Medicine, 12,* 45–55.

Krieger, D. T., Allen, W., Rizzo, F., & Krieger, H. P. (1971). Characterization of the normal temporal pattern of plasma corticosteroid levels. *Journal of Clinical Endocrinology and Metabolism, 32,* 266–284.

Kripke, D. F. (1976). Serotonin depression. *Science, 194,* 214.

Lapin, I. P., & Oxenkrug, G. F. (1969). Intensification of the central serotoninergic processes as a possible determinant of the thymoleptic effect. *Lancet 1,* 132–136.

Loosen, P. T., & Prange, A. J. (1982). Serum thyrotropin response to the thyrotropin-releasing hormone in psychiatric patients: A review. *American Journal of Psychiatry, 139,* 405–416.

Loosen, P. T., Prange, A. J., & Wilson, I. C. (1978). Influence of cortisol on TRH-induced TSH response in depression. *American Journal of Psychiatry, 135,* 244–246.

Maas, J. W. (1975). Biogenic amines and depression: Biochemical and pharmacological separation of two types of depression. *Archives of General Psychiatry, 32,* 1357–1361.

Maas, J. W., Fawcett, J. A., & Dekirmenjian, H. (1968). 3-Methoxy-4-hydroxyphenylglycol (MHPG) excretion in depressive states: A pilot study. *Archives of General Psychiatry, 19,* 129–134.

Maas, J. W., Fawcett, J. A., Dekirmenjian, H. (1972). Catecholamine metabolism, depressive illness, and drug response. *Archives of General Psychiatry, 26,* 252–262.

Maas, J. W., Hattox, S. E., Greene, N. M., & Landis, D. H. (1979). 3-Methoxy-4-hydroxyphenyleneglycol production by human brain in vivo. *Science, 205,* 1025–1027.

Maas, J. W., Kocsis, J. H., Bowden, C. L., Davis, J. M., Redmond, D. E., Hanin, I., & Robins, E. (1982). Pretreatment neurotransmitter metabolites and response to imipramine or amitriptyline treatment. *Psychological Medicine, 12,* 37–43.

Maas, J W., & Landis, D. H. (1971). The metabolism of circulating norepinephrine in human subjects. *Journal of Pharmacology and Experimental Therapeutics, 177,* 600–612.

Mardh, G., Sjoquist, B., & Anggard, E. (1981). Norepinephrine metabolism in man using deuterium labelling: The conversion of 4-hydroxy-3-methoxyphenylglycol to 4-hydroxy-3-methoxymandelic acid. *Journal of Neurochemistry, 36,* 1181–1185.

Martin, J. B., Reichlin, S., & Brown, G. M. (1977). *Clinical neuroendocrinology.* Philadelphia: FA Davis Company.

Mendels, J., & Frazer, A. (1975). Reduced central serotonergic activity in mania: Implications for the relationship between depression and mania. *British Journal of Psychiatry, 126,* 241–248.

Murphy, D. L., Brodie, H. K. H., Goodwin, F. K., & Bunney, W. E. (1971). Regular induction of hypomania by L-dopa in "bipolar" manic-depressive patients. *Nature, 229,* 135–136.

Murphy, D. L., Campbell, I., & Costa, J. L. (1978). Current status of the indoleamine hypothesis of affective disorders. In M. A. Lipton, A. DiMascio, & K. F. Killam (Eds.), *Psychopharmacology: A generation of progress* (pp. 1235–1247). New York: Raven Press.

Murphy, D. L., Goodwin, F. K., Brodie, H. K. H., & Bunney, W. E. (1973). L-dopa, dopamine, and hypomania. *American Journal of Psychiatry, 130,* 79–82.

Murphy, G. E., Woodruff, R. A., Herjanic, M., & Super, G. (1974). Variability of the clinical course of primary affective disorder. *Archives of General Psychiatry, 30,* 757–761.

Ostrow, D. G., Pandey, G. N., Davis, J. M., Hurt, S. W., & Tosteson, D. C. (1978). A heritable disorder of lithium transport in erythrocytes of a subpopulation of manic-depressive patients. *American Journal of Psychiatry, 135,* 1370–1378.

Ostrow, D. G., Trevisan, M., Okonek, A., Gibbons, R., Cooper, R., & Davis, J. M. (1982). Sodium dependent membrane processes in major affective disorders. In E. Usdin & I. Hanin (Eds.), *Biological markers in psychiatry and neurology* (pp. 153–168). Oxford: Pergamon Press.

Potkin, S. G., Wyatt, R. J., & Karoum, F. (1980). Phenylethylamine (PEA) and phenylacetic acid (PAA) in the urine of chronic schizophrenic patients and controls. *Psychopharmacology Bulletin, 16,* 52–54.

Prange, A. J., Wilson, I. C., Lara, P. P., Alltop, L. B., & Breese, G. R. (1972). Effects of thyrotropin-releasing hormone in depression. *Lancet, 2,* 999–1002.

Prange, A. J., Wilson, I. C., Lynn, C. W., Alltop, L. B., & Stikeleather, R. A. (1974). L-tryptophan in mania: Contribution to a permissive hypothesis of affective disorders. *Archives of General Psychiatry, 30,* 56–62.

Randrup, A., & Braestrup, C. (1977). Uptake inhibition of biogenic amines by newer antidepressant drugs: Relevance to the dopamine hypothesis of depression. *Psychopharmacology, 53,* 309–314.

Randrup, A., Munkvad, I., Fog, R., Gerlach, J., Molander, L., Kjellberg, B., & Scheel-Kruger, J. (1975). Mania, depression, and brain dopamine. In W. B. Essman & L. Valzelli (Eds.), *Current developments in psychopharmacology* (Vol. 2) (pp. 206–248). New York: Spectrum Publications.

Risch, S. C., Kalin, N. H., & Murphy, D. L. (1982). Neurochemical mechanisms in the affective disorders and neuroendocrine correlates. *Journal of Clinical Psychopharmacology, 1,* 180–185.

Rubin, R. T., & Mandell, A. J. (1966). Adrenal cortical activity in pathological emotional states: A review. *American Journal of Psychiatry, 123,* 387–400.

Sabelli, H. C., Fawcett, J., Gusovsky, F., Edwards, J., Jeffriess, H., & Javaid, J. (1983a). Phenylacetic acid as an indicator in bipolar affective disorders. *Journal of Clinical Psychopharmacology, 3,* 268–270.

Sabelli, H. C., Fawcett, J., Gusovsky, F., Javaid, J., Edwards, J., & Jeffriess, H. (1983b). Urinary phenyl acetate: A diagnostic test for depression? *Science, 220,* 1187–1188.

Sabelli, H. C., Fawcett, J., Javaid, J. I., & Bagri, S. (1983c). The methylphenidate test for differentiating desipramine-responsive from nortriptyline-responsive depression. *American Journal of Psychiatry, 140,* 212–214.

Sabelli, H. C., & Mosnaim, A. D. (1974). Phenylethylamine hypothesis of affective behavior. *American Journal of Psychiatry, 131,* 695–699.

Sachar, E. J., Hellman, L., Roffwarg, H., Halpern, F. S., Fukushima, D. K., & Gallagher, T. F. (1973). Disrupted 24-hour patterns of cortisol secretion in psychotic depression. *Archives of General Psychiatry, 28,* 19–24.

Sandler, M., Ruthven, C. R. J., Goodwin, B. L., & Coppen, A. (1979). *Clinica Chimica Acta, 93,* 169–171.

Schanberg, S. M., Breese, G. R., Schildkraut, J. J., Gordon, E. K., & Kopin, I. J. (1968). 3-Methoxy-4-hydroxyphenylglycol sulfate in brain and cerebrospinal fluid. *Biochemical Pharmacology, 17,* 2006–2008.

Schatzberg, A. F., Orsulak, P. J., Rosenbaum, A. H., Maruta, T., Kruger, E. R., Cole, J. O., & Schildkraut, J. J. (1980). Toward a biochemical classification of depressive disorders. IV. Pretreatment urinary MHPG levels as predictors of antidepressant response to imipramine. *Communications in Psychopharmacology, 4,* 441–445.

Schatzberg, A. F., Rosenbaum, A. H., Orsulak, P. J., Rohde, W. A., Maruta, T., Kruger, E. R., Cole, J. O., & Schildkraut, J. J. (1981). Toward a biochemical classification of depressive disorders. III. Pretreatment urinary MHPG levels as predictors of response to treatment with maprotiline. *Psychopharmacology, 75,* 34–38.

Schildkraut, J. J. (1965). The catecholamine hypothesis of affective disorders: A review of supporting evidence. *American Journal of Psychiatry, 122,* 509–522.

Schildkraut, J. J., Orsulak, P. J., Schatzberg, A. F., Cole, J. O., & Rosenbaum, A. H. (1981). Possible pathophysiological mechanisms in subtypes of unipolar depressive disorders based on differences in urinary MHPG levels. *Psychopharmacology Bulletin, 17,* 90–91.

Schildkraut, J. J., Orsulak, P. J., Schatzberg, A. F., Gudeman, J. E., Cole, J. O., Rohde, W. A., & LaBrie, R. A. (1978). Toward a biochemical classification of depressive disorders. I. Differences in urinary excretion of MHPG and other catecholamine metabolites in clinically defined subtypes of depression. *Archives of General Psychiatry, 35,* 1427–1433.

Siever, L., Insel, T., & Uhde, T. (1982). Noradrenergic challenges in the affective disorders. *Journal of Clinical Psychopharmacology, 1*, 193–206.

Spitzer, R. L., Endicott, J., & Robins, E. (1978a). *Research diagnostic criteria.* New York: New York State Psychiatric Institute.

Spitzer, R. L., Endicott, J., & Robins, E. (1978b). Research Diagnostic Criteria: Rationale and reliability. *Archives of General Psychiatry, 35*, 773–782.

Sternbach, H., Gwirtsman, H., & Gerner, R. H. (1981). The dexamethasone suppression test and response to methylphenidate in depression. *American Journal of Psychiatry, 138*, 1629–1631.

Sulser, F. (1982). Antidepressant drug research: Its impact on neurobiology and psychobiology. *Advances in Biochemical Psychopharmacology, 31*, 1–20.

Sulser, F., Vetulani, J., & Mobley, P. L. (1978). Mode of action of antidepressant drugs. *Biochemical Pharmacology, 27*, 257–261.

Sweeney, D. R., Maas, J. W., & Heninger, G. R. (1978). State anxiety, physical activity, and urinary 3-methoxy-4-hydroxyphenethylene glycol excretion. *Archives of General Psychiatry, 35*, 1418–1423.

Targum, S. D. (1983). Neuroendocrine challenge studies in clinical psychiatry. *Psychiatric Annals, 13*, 385–395.

Targum, S. D., Sullivan, A. C., & Byrnes, S. M. (1982). Neuroendocrine interrelationships in major depressive disorders. *American Journal of Psychiatry, 139*, 282–286.

Van Kammen, D. P., & Murphy, D. L. (1975). Attenuation of the euphoriant and activating effects of d- and l-amphetamine by lithium carbonate treatment. *Psychopharmacologia, 44*, 215–224.

Van Kammen, D. P., & Murphy, D. L. (1978). Prediction of imipramine antidepressant response by a one-day d-amphetamine trial. *American Journal of Psychiatry, 135*, 1179–1184.

Van Kammen, D. P., & Murphy, D. L. (1979). Prediction of antidepressant response to lithium carbonate by a 1-day administration of d-amphetamine in unipolar depressed women. *Neuropsychobiology, 5*, 266–273.

Van Praag, H. M. (1981). Management of depression with serotonin precursors. *Biological Psychiatry, 16*, 291–310.

Veith, R. C., Bielski, R. J., Bloom, V., Fawcett, J. A., Narasimhachari, N., & Friedel, R. O. (1983). Urinary MHPG excretion and treatment with desipramine or amitriptyline: Prediction of response, effect of treatment, and methodological hazards. *Journal of Clinical Psychopharmacology, 3*, 18–27.

Vetulani, J., & Sulser, F. (1975). Action of various antidepressant treatments reduces reactivity of noradrenergic cyclic AMP-generating system in limbic forebrain. *Nature, 257*, 495–496.

Wehr, T. A., Muscettola, G., & Goodwin, F. K. (1980). Urinary 3-methoxy-4-hydroxyphenyglycol circadian rhythm: Early timing (phase-advance) in manic-depressives compared with normal subjects. *Archives of General Psychiatry, 37*, 257–263.

Weissman, M. M., & Klerman, G. L. (1977). The chronic depressive in the community: Unrecognized and poorly treated. *Comprehensive Psychiatry, 18*, 523–532.

Weissman, M. M., & Myers, J. K. (1978a). Rates and risks of depressive symptoms in a United States urban community. *Acta Psychiatrica Scandinavica, 57*, 219–231.

Weissman, M. M., & Myers, J. K. (1978b). Affective disorders in a US urban community: The use of Research Diagnostic Criteria in an epidemiological survey. *Archives of General Psychiatry, 35,* 1304–1311.

Weissman, M. M., Myers, J. K., & Harding, P. S. (1978). Psychiatric disorders in a US urban community: 1975–1976. *American Journal of Psychiatry, 135,* 459–462.

Whybrow, P. C., & Prange, A. J. (1981). A hypothesis of thyroid-catecholamine-receptor interaction: Its relevance to affective illness. *Archives of General Psychiatry, 38,* 106–113.

Zis, A. P., & Goodwin, F. K. (1979). Novel antidepressants and the biogenic amine hypothesis of depression: The case for iprindole and mianserin. *Archives of General Psychiatry, 36,* 1097–1107.

Zis, A. P., & Goodwin, F. K. (1982). The amine hypothesis. In E. S. Paykel (Ed.), *Handbook of affective disorders* (pp. 175–190). New York: Guilford Press.

	Short-Term
	Hospitalization and
3	the Depressed Patient
	Kathleen Ryan Delaney

Short-term psychiatric units operate on specific goals. They aim for rapid improvement of patients' symptoms and attempt to return patients to their home settings and former lifestyles. These goals are accomplished through somatic and professional therapies, medications, and strategic utilization of the hospital environment and milieu staff. While goals are clear, debate continues on why any particular milieu or treatment approach is effective in helping patients achieve these aims (Greenhill, 1979; Herz, 1972). In fact, Erickson's (1975) review of outcome research conducted in psychiatric hospitals concluded that questions of what works, why, and with whom remain largely unanswered.

The ambiguity surrounding the effectiveness of interventions is of particular concern to nurses caring for depressed patients. Since there exists a problem of demonstrating the worth of treatment on short-term units, nurses roles and functions also come into question. Typically, nurses hold key positions in coordinating treatment on short-term units. They execute a treatment approach that advocates groups, activities, and a structured day to benefit patients. This milieu therapy approach recognizes the potential of the environment to help patients. However, a search of the literature reveals little direct evidence to show this organization of care is beneficial over other treatment structures (Perrow, 1965).

The majority of milieu therapy research focuses on patients' perceptions of the tone of the unit and staff attitudes that contribute to a positive atmosphere

NURSING INTERVENTIONS IN DEPRESSION   Copyright © 1985 by Grune & Stratton, Inc.
ISBN 0-8089-1710-2   All rights of reproduction in any form reserved.

(Edelson & Paul, 1977; Ellsworth & Maroney, 1972; Moos, 1968; Moos & Schwartz, 1972; Weinstein, 1979). These studies describe the dimensions of a therapeutic milieu but not how to bring about the desired qualities. Indeed, several authors agree that milieu therapy is an ideology that lacks an actual technology (Abroms, 1969; Rasinski, et al., 1980; Sills, 1975). Professionals know *what* milieu treatment is but not *how* to institute it. This lack of defined methods leaves nurses coordinating treatment on the units with more of a tradition of care followed over the years rather than specific interventions substantiated by research.

Recently, the author completed a research project that responds to the need for clarification of treatment methods on short-term psychiatric units (Delaney, 1984). The research aimed at determining why certain aspects of hospitalization were therapeutic. To find the answer, psychiatric patients were asked to discuss their illnesses, specific therapies, professional relationships, and finally, how they viewed discharge and discharge readiness. The purpose of the research interview was to discover the *why* of patients' responses to treatment. In essence, patients described how they saw themselves utilizing psychiatric care.

THE RESEARCH PROCESS

In this study, 50 patients were interviewed, 80% of whom were depressed. They were hospitalized on two short-term psychiatric units where a similar approach in treatment was instituted. Both units stressed a multidisciplinary approach and the use of a therapeutic milieu, and both structured the patients' days around various groups and activities. Over a 6-month period of data collection, 350 hours of participant observation occurred along with the 50 unstructured interviews.

Throughout the research, the emphasis was on discovering patient's perceptions of treatment, and of learning how these perceptions evolved. The value of such a focus has been supported by symbolic interaction theory, which is based on the idea that individuals develop personalized viewpoints on any given situation; e.g., each person has his or her own unique perspective on the role the family plays in one's ongoing lifestyle. Interactionists stipulate that once one understands how people see particular situations, the logic behind their actions is revealed. It therefore seemed appropriate to design this study in line with interactionist thought; in other words, to understand patients' behavior by learning how they explain and define their illnesses as well as the important events in their lives.

The Concept of Control

During the data analysis, it became apparent that patients were struggling to build confidence in their ability to function after discharge. Most respondents had recently experienced a disruption in their lives, challenging them to put their lives (moods, thoughts, and emotions) back into equilibrium. What patients said about how their lives had changed was organized around the idea of control. The disruption or change patients described was thought of as a loss of control and the patients' notions of recovery as regaining control. Learning how patients saw themselves regaining control of their lives clarified why they had responded in a particular way to the treatment program. Essentially, patients viewed hospitalization as helpful if somewhere in its offerings there was an intervention that fit with their plans for regaining control.

The following case example illustrates how a patients' perceptions of illness and recovery can be organized around the concept of control and, further, how a patient's definition of achieving control determined what elements of treatment were regarded as beneficial.

Case example. S., a 74-year-old woman hospitalized for depression, described her problems as sleeplessness, anxiety, and depression. This was her second hospitalization, her first was eight months earlier after experiencing a half-year of insomnia and depression. Upon discharge from this first hospital stay, S. immediately began to be troubled with sleeplessness and anxiety. The experience of discharge followed by an immediate return of her symptoms became an important factor in how she defined control. In order to have a sense of control, S. had to believe that she could regulate sleep. During much of the interview, S. focused on the fear of insomnia returning after discharge. She was determined to prevent that, explaining her plans in the following words:

I could have gone home Wednesday, but I wanted to stay until Friday because I've got to establish a sleep pattern. This is what helped bring about my downfall and tore me apart. That brought on the depression, not sleeping nights. I've worked out a schedule where I take a pill at the time I go to bed. I'm taking one pill called _____; it's more or less a relaxant, a tranquilizer. I go to bed at 10:30. I'm up again at maybe around 12 or 12:30, then go to the bathroom and fall asleep. I'm up again at about 5:30 which is wonderful, even it I get 4 or 5 hours. Older people don't sleep as much as young people (Interview 22, Delaney, 1984)

This statement shows that S. believed lack of sleep actually caused her depression. Therefore, it was understandable that sleep became her central control issue and a crucial component in her process of recovery. In the previous statement, S. outlined her plan to regain a sense of control. With the help of medication, she established a schedule for her nights. She also redefined what constituted a good night's sleep: just 4–5 hours of rest. Through these plans and redefinitions, S. ceased to be a victim of insomnia and learned to control her sleep.

S. valued hospitalization because through it she regained the confidence that she could go home and sleep at night. She cited particular aspects of treatment as helpful since they helped her establish a sleep pattern. For instance, S. said it was crucial that staff members understood the ramifications of her insomnia and agreed with her goal of establishing a sleep pattern. She was uncomfortable during her previous hospitalization because staff discounted her concern for sleep. S. needed to believe others empathized with her problem, but perceived groups and activities as inconsequential in the process of establishing a sleep pattern. She thought the topics discussed in groups had nothing to do with her problems and dismissed them as "not my interest." Throughout the research interview, S.'s evaluation of hospitalization became meaningful in the context of her emphasis on regaining control of sleep.

It is difficult to define how hospitalization helps any particular patient or patient group since each patient's endorsement of disillusionment with the hospital is rooted in particular circumstances and definitions. What is essential, however, is that broad statements about hospital use can be drawn out of the perceptions that patients share over loss of control and methods of regaining control. Following are patients' ideas on how their need for control influenced their responses to hospitalization. Although patients develop many strategies for regaining control, three common methods emerged in the course of this research study: medication, self-definitions, and self-understanding.

Medication as a Cure

During the research interviews, 20 patients said hospitalization helped them regain a sense of control. Of these 20 patients, 8 defined control in terms of ridding themselves of depression, maintaining they were in the hospital to be cured. For this cure they depended on either medication or Electric Convulsive Therapy (ECT). These patients resisted discussions on the background of their depressions. In their view, medication would cure their depressions and talking about feelings or life situations was useless. One such patient reacted to his illness by refusing to think about why his depression occurred, claiming it came on him "in mysterious ways," and saying the doctor would engineer a cure through ECT. This patient had reason to expect such a recovery. In his one previous psychiatric hospitalization he received ECT, went home, and had no symptom of depression for 4 years. He anticipated the same result from this hospital stay.

Because they believed in a cure through ECT and medication, the 8 patients dismissed other types of interventions. Because of their denial that depressions involved problems in their life styles or relationships, they saw no need for groups and talking therapies. These patients separated their illnesses and hospital experiences from other life events. They expected to be rid of depression, go home, and live their lives as if hospitalization had not occurred.

Maintaining a Particular Self-Definition

The majority of patients interviewed said their loss of control came from depressions, situational problems, or thought disorders. In most cases, regaining control involved talking out their problems or a medication cure. Nine patients differed in how they defined illness and recovery: they deemphasized both their depressions and need for psychiatric help, and did not associate regaining control with resolving their depressions. Rather, they linked control with returning home to a place or lifestyle in which they felt comfortable. While hospitalized, they maintained a sense of control by preserving their self-definitions as individuals without psychiatric conditions.

For example, M., an elderly woman admitted for depression, said she did not know why her husband and doctor insisted on hospitalization. M. acknowledged that since retirement she spent most of her day sleeping, but saw nothing unusual about this behavior. In her mind, thyroid testing was the only reason for hospitalization. Since M. defined treatment as a medical workup, she resisted involvement in the therapy program, remaining in her room between tests. Her only goal was to return home.

Like M., these patients stayed apart from peers and staff and limited their participation in the milieu program. They refused to define themselves as mental patients, seeing themselves as healthy individuals. During the research interview they frequently depicted groups and activities as stigmatizing—something for patients with mental problems. So rather than gain control through treatment, hospitalization represented a negative identity and an alteration in their self-definition. For these nine patients control would come once they were home and back to a particular lifestyle and comfortable identity.

Control through Self-Understanding

Twelve of the 50 patients interviewed said getting better meant improving one's coping, attitudes, or communication style. They connected their psychiatric conditions to their life styles, relationships, and behavior patterns. For example, one man believed that his depression occurred because of the multiple stresses in his life. Recently he had moved from his home, leaving friends and family behind. Hopes and expectations for his new employment had fallen. For him regaining control demanded sorting through his response to recent life changes. He viewed therapy as helpful in this process. The 12 patients also saw themselves utilizing the insight derived from therapy to regain control. Groups and relationships with staff were important. The patients searched for feedback, input, and support. They believed treatment helped them sort through problems and learn to deal with stress. One woman described her experience in group in the following way:

I was better able to understand my problems through group meetings, which were very, very helpful. They not only allowed me to talk about my situation in complete confidentiality, but I also found elements of my own problems in other people's circumstances. They were dealing with some of the things I was dealing with. Well, my feeling was, I was able to talk about these things and it's not just me in an apartment building. (Interview 35, Delaney, 1984)

This patient was attempting to cope with a recent injury and subsequent changes in her life style. She valued group therapy for the opportunity to discuss her problems and for support and feedback from other patients. In a sense, she and the other individuals in this group were the ideal patients—utilizing treatment in the way it was designed to function.

Patients Who Did Not Regain Control

Fifteen patients in this study reported they had not regained a sense of control in their lives. Nine of these patients optimistically believed they would *eventually* regain control after discharge, while the other six expressed pessimism, seeing little hope for relief from their depressions and emotional turmoil. The pessimistic patients reported needing to be prepared for a life of anguish; two of these patients considered suicide. Reasons for desperate feelings included physical problems, significant losses, and fear of the emotional illness becoming chronically out of control.

The pessismistic group said hospitalization offered little help. For some, the hospital represented an unreality of warmth and relationships that faded after discharge. Others saw treatment as a long struggle and wondered if they had the strength to continue. One similarity between these six patients was that although they saw little hope for the future, they rejected health professionals' suggestions for treatment. They preferred to go home, try to struggle through life, or end it as they saw fit.

The nine optimistic patients also rejected health professionals' possible solutions to their problems. However, they hoped that eventually one would surface. One such woman interviewed with the author during her second psychiatric hospitalization. After her first admission, A. left the hospital symptom-free. The second time, A.'s physician suggested her depression was recurrent and she may have to learn to live with a certain amount of symptomology. Her physician's conclusion disturbed A. because of head pains that accompanied her depressions. She rejected the idea of recurring depression because living with the head pains was intolerable to her. Unwilling to accept the physician's prognosis, A. believed a drug combination would eventually control her depressive symptoms. Once she was discharged, she intended to consult other psychiatrists and find a pharmacological solution.

Patients like A. presented a paradoxical response to hospitalization. They perceived a need for psychiatric treatment, were quite desperate for admission, and remained in the hospital for 3 weeks or longer. Yet, when they looked back on their hospitalization during the research interview, they expressed dissatisfaction with their progress. At the root of this dissatisfaction was a desire to achieve a certain level of symptom resolution, that, given their circumstances, was not readily attainable. In their view, hospitalization had not provided the help they anticipated. Afraid that once they were at home the symptoms would reappear, however, the patients often remained in the hospital, while trying to find other solutions to their problems.

The important thing the hospital offered was time. Not ready to face what seemed to be insurmountable situations at home, patients viewed the hospital as a sanctuary, and perceived extending their hospital stay as an opportunity to improve their level of functioning, or perhaps change circumstances at home. One man, J., suffered both depression and spinal arthritis. Physicians suggested J. focus on his depression, because, in their opinion, J.'s arthritic pain increased when his depression deepened. J. believed psychiatry was an "ascientific" profession and mistrusted its methods. The physicians recommended outpatient psychiatric care that J.'s family demanded he attend. J. was not willing to follow this recommendation and remained in the hospital, hoping to find another way of dealing with his pain and depression.

On the positive side, the hospital offered support. Several patients reported feeling alienated and alone outside the hospital. They were ashamed of having emotional problems, and felt that significant others were failing to empathize with their depressions. In the hospital, and particularly with the nursing staff, they found a group of individuals who understood their experience. As was true of many of the patients interviewed, they counted on nurses to care and cited them as a valued component of their hospital stay.

Summary

This section has focused on underlying themes in patients' definitions of control. How patients come to define control as a complete cure of their psychiatric conditions, how some patients connect control to resolution of emotional turmoil, and finally, how some come to associate control with a particular lifestyle and self-definition was demonstrated. Patients who viewed control as eventual because of an unwillingness to accept a partial solution to their problems were described. The key point is how patients view treatment in relation to their need to restore a sense of control in their lives. What nurses can do for patients really depends on each individual patient's definition of illness, recovery, and treatment, and how they see themselves regaining a sense of control in their lives.

NURSING IMPLICATIONS

Nurses might use the previous information in a variety of ways. Below are four suggestions.

Use of patients' perceptions.   First, the findings of this study indicate the value of understanding patients' definitions of control and regaining control. The idea of control is a way to organize what patients say about illness and recovery. Translating patients' perspectives into a control framework is a process. By listening to what patients say about their lives, one starts to understand their values; what is crucial to their self esteem, what role in life they emphasize, and essentially, how they define themselves.

When allowed to control the agenda of a conversation, patients usually will reveal what is crucial to them: they will narrate a key event or story to help make themselves understood. Key events might be connected to their career, upbringing, or important relationships. Within each patient's "story" lies their control issue.

During data collection, an example of a patient's "story" was recorded in the following field note:

G. began the interview by relating that for 20 years doctors said she was schizophrenic, but now she was diagnosed as manic depressive. During this hospitalization the doctor told her she could take Lithium and be able to function. She mentioned repeatedly that if she took Lithium, she would be able to take care of herself. It was difficult to understand the full ramifications of Lithium and the new diagnosis until G. discussed living in a nursing home. With great detail G. described how she moved to a nursing home when her daughter could no longer care for her. *The move to a nursing home was the key event.* As the interview progressed it was apparent how this central issue tied together many other aspects of G.'s story. One quote gave the symbolic link, "Now since I am taking my Lithium I will be able to wait on myself; that's why I don't want to go back to a nursing home." G's control issue was not her psychiatric condition but moving back with her daughter. There was an urgency for me to understand what it was like living in a nursing home. G. seemed to be saying if you are going to understand me, you have to understand this (Field note 109, Delaney, 1984)

The above story helped the author to understand why G. derived such hope from treatment. As with G., patients' stories provided a context for the rest of the interview, and as a result, meanings of other responses became apparent. By listening and understanding how patients are describing their lives, it is possible to distill what aspects of the patient's life are crucial to his or her sense of control and what occurred to prompt loss of control. Losing control does not necessarily occur because of the onset of a psychiatric condition: a change in life style imposed on the patient, aging, physical illness, pain might be a key control issue. When the nurse listens to patients and relates back what the patients are saying about life and control, it is then possible to explore how patients see themselves restoring control in their lives and how treatment fits into these plans.

While discussions with patients should be basically unstructured, allowing their perspectives to emerge, the nurse hopes to gather information covering certain topic areas. Here are examples of questions that should be addressed during the course of assessment interviews:

• What happened in patients' lives to cause them to come to the hospital?
• What has to happen to give the patients a sense of control in their lives?
• What do patients tell themselves about why depression occurred?

- What are patients doing in treatment that will help them regain control?
- How do patients come to think of recovery in this manner?
- Why or why not are groups and activities helpful to patients?
- How do patients see the nursing staff's job, and the physician's role?
- What are patients' plans for maintaining stability after discharge?

From this type of information one can formulate how patients define important aspects of their lives and how treatment and the illness experience have been integrated into these definitions. This information can provide a starting point for discussions on a patient's belief system. The focus is on patients' self-definitions and what involvement in treatment means to them. It is particularly helpful with patients who are reluctant to talk about themselves or become involved in a relationship. With a resistive patient, one avoids a discussion centered on compliance issues, and instead the relationship begins to build around an understanding of the patient's viewpoint. Patients then experience talking to someone who is trying to understand instead of trying to impose a contrary viewpoint.

Recognition of patients' belief systems.   A second nursing implication involves expectations for patients' participation in the milieu. In most psychiatric hospitals, milieu refers to the tone of the unit and the predictable nature of the environment. Milieu treatment is the schedule of groups and activities that order the patients' days. In these groups it is assumed that patients will do some internal work, perhaps analyzing their behavior or exploring feelings.

Patients in this study reported they did not necessarily use groups or the milieu for these reasons. Patients said the hospital served a variety of purposes, e.g., as a sanctuary from stress, a place to recover while medications began to ease depression, or as a break from family expectations. Currently, the psychiatric hospital staff operate as if the patient population held a homogenous belief system on hospital treatment and the way to recover. In addition, staff seem to believe that all patients will eventually see the value of talk therapy and insight. In reality there are multiple beliefs on ways to use the hospital. Thus, professionals responsible for planning psychiatric programs should avoid designing milieu groups around how they hope patients will think and react; rather, groups and activities should adapt to the variety of belief systems.

A more flexible approach to treatment planning is needed, one which accounts for patients' definitions of treatment, illness, and recovery. Patients may define control in terms of mastery over pain, role adjustment, or resolving family turmoil. Alternately, patients may remain in the hospital unwilling to accept professional help, defining control in terms of securing a discharge. Nurses must be able to shift frameworks when addressing these various definitions of regaining control.

Groups should be formed to address configurations of patients and belief systems. In this case, group content would be flexible, depending on a particular patient mix. For example, groups can be organized around several older patients all struggling to adjust to aging. If there are patients who do not see the need for hospitalization, but remain in the facility, they can group together and explore their self-definitions and how they see themselves reacting to the label of mental illness. A group of chronically ill patients would benefit from a discussion group on how to survive in a halfway house, or more generally, how to adjust to the role of a chronic mental patient. The important thing is to acknowledge and explore these varying definitions of recovery and control and avoid operating a milieu as if a homogenous belief system of illness and recovery existed among patients.

Concept of caring.   During the research interviews, patients talked about experiencing the acute symptoms of depression. As they described living through a depression, they told of their sufferings; the jitters on the inside, the need to constantly move, and having time pass slowly, so slowly that patients hurried to sleep to relieve depression. Against this backdrop of suffering, patients perceived relatives and neighbors as unempathetic with their problems. Families often told patients to try harder or to "snap out" of their depressions.

Patients expressed a need to have someone who understood their depressions; nurses were frequently identified as this source of support. Even when patients were using hospitalization to receive medications, they expressed the need to have contact with someone who cared. Often seemingly insignificant interactions with nurses made patients feel cared for and understood. Here is how one patient described staff support.

I remember there was a thunderstorm. I was so scared. I was having dreams and still thinking everything had something to do with me. At one clap of thunder I just went racing out of my room. S. (a staff member) caught me and he said "Do you need to talk; I have time." I said, "No," but having him there helped. (Interview 6, Delaney, 1984)

For several weeks of hospitalization this patient was frightened and unsure of herself. Staff's caring was both reassuring and comforting.

As professionals, nurses need to recognize and explore this vital function. They may be underestimating the import of this human element of the profession. Nurses are in a key position to offer this support to patients, to understand their world. As a first step, nurses should conceptualize how a tone of caring is established both within a relationship and on the unit.

Understanding patients' biological perspective.   The final nursing implication involves the issue of medication. Findings of this study indicate patients relied on antidepressant medication to varying degrees (Delaney, 1984). Some patients thought medications eased their depressions, while others depended on medication for a cure. Believing medication would bring about biological normality, some patients de-emphasized the role of talk therapy in regaining control. Because of this strong belief in the power of medication they also tended to dismiss the psychological component of their illnesses or the emotional impact of their depressions.

Research is needed to discover what nurses can offer patients who feel they are in the hospital in order to wait for medications to work. On one hand nurses need to recognize a belief in medication, especially when other professionals are laboring to build patients' confidence in the effectiveness of antidepressants; on the other hand are nurses' professional beliefs in the impact of illness on self, and the need to open up patients' self-awareness.

To strike a balance between these two belief systems, nurses need to clarify what they can offer biologically oriented patients. One way to gather information is to conduct exit interviews with patients, asking specifically what was helpful about the hospital and what was lacking. In this research project, such interviews were a rich source of information. This type of feedback is needed, not to gather praise or criticism, but to learn how to coordinate medication with psychologically oriented therapies and treatment approaches. Once nursing and allied professions are clear on the mesh of medication and milieu, patients can begin to understand how to use milieu therapy while maintaining confidence in medication.

SUMMARY

These previous suggestions are a start in integrating patients' perspectives into treatment planning on short-term psychiatric units. All conclusions were based on what patients said about their hospital experiences and how they defined illness and recovery. The use of patients' perspectives should not be isolated to research studies. They are a vital source of information and a means of evaluating nursing care. Patients' perspectives should be understood and used in communicating with patients and planning care. This would be a step, not towards involving patients in their own care, but towards involving nurses in patients' perceptions of the recovery process.

REFERENCES

Abroms, G. M. (1969). Defining milieu therapy. *Archives of General Psychiatry, 21,* 553–560.

Delaney, K. R. (1984). Patients' perceptions of the significance of treatment on short-term psychiatric units. *Dissertation Abstracts International, 44,* 3037B. (University Microfilms No. DA 840 1780)

Edelson, R. J., & Paul, G. L. (1977). Staff "attitude" and "atmosphere" scores as a function of ward size and patient chronicity. *Journal of Consulting and Clinical Psychology, 45,* 874–884.

Ellsworth, R., & Maroney, R. (1972). Characteristics of psychiatric programs and their effects on patients adjustment. *Journal of Consulting and Clinical Psychology, 39,* 436–447.

Erickson, R. C. (1975). Outcome studies in mental hospitals: A review. *Psychological Bulletin, 82,* 519–540.

Grenhill, M. H. (1979). Psychiatric units in general hospital: 1979. *Hospital and Community Psychiatry, 30,* 169–182.

Herz, M. I. (1972). The therapeutic community: A critique. *Hospital and Community Psychiatry, 23,* 69–72.

Moos, R. (1968). Situational analysis of a therapeutic community milieu. *Journal of Abnormal Psychology, 73,* 49–61.

Moos, R., & Schwartz, J. (1972). Treatment environment and treatment outcome. *Journal of Mental and Nervous Disease, 154,* 264–275.

Perrow, C. (1965). Hospitals: technology, structure, and goals. In J. G. March (Eds.), *Handbook of Organizations* (pp. 910–971). Chicago: Rand McNally.

Rasinski, K., Rozensky, R., & Pasulka, P. (1980). Practical implications of a theory of the "therapeutic milieu" for psychiatric nursing practice. *JPN and Mental Health Services, 8,* 16–29.

Sills, G. (1978). Use of milieu therapy. In F. L. Huey (Ed.), *Psychiatric Nursing from 1946 to 1974: A Report on the State of the Art,* (pp. 23–35). New York: American Journal of Nursing Company.

Weinstein, R. M. (1979). Patient attitudes toward mental hospitalization: A review of quantitative research. *Journal of Health and Social Behavior, 20,* 237–258.

SUGGESTED READINGS

Allen, J. C., & Barton, G. M. (1976). Patients' comments about hospitalization: implications for changes. *Comprehensive Psychiatry, 17,* 631–640.

Almond, R., Kensiston, K., & Boltax, S. (1968). The value system of a milieu therapy unit. *Archives of General Psychiatry, 19,* 545–561.

Almond, R., Keniston, K., & Boltax, S. (1969). Patient value change in milieu therapy. *Archives of General Psychiatry, 20,* 339–351.

Brady, J. P., Zeller, W. W., & Rezenkoff, M. (1959). Attitudinal factors influencing outcome of treatment of hospitalized psychiatric patients. *Journal of Clinical and Experimental Psychopathology, 20,* 326–334.

Goldstein, R. H., Cittone, R. A., Dressler, D., Racy, J., & Willis, J. (1972). What benefits patients? An inquiry into the opinions of psychiatric inpatients and their residents. *Psychiatric Quarterly, 46,* 49–80.

Gould, E., & Glick, I. D. (1976). Patient–staff judgment of treatment program helpfulness on a psychiatric ward. *British Journal of Medical Psychology, 49,* 23–33.

Gynther, M. D., Rezinkoff, M., & Fishman, M. (1963). Attitudes of psychiatric patients towards treatment, psychiatrists, and mental hospitals. *Journal of Nervous and Mental Disease, 136,* 68–71.

Jones, N. F., & Kahn, M. W. (1964). Patient attitudes as related to social class and other variables concerning hospitalization. *Journal of Consulting Psychology, 28,* 403–408.

Jones, N. F., Kahn, M. W., & Macdonald, J. M. (1963). Psychiatric patients' views of mental illness, hospitalization, and treatment. *Journal of Nervous and Mental Disease, 136,* 82–87.

Kaplan, H. B., Boyd, I., & Bloon, S. W. (1964). Patient culture and the evaluation of self. *Psychiatry, 27,* 116–126.

Lee, H. S. (1979). Patients' comments on psychiatric inpatient treatment experiences: Patient–therapist relationships and their implications for treatment outcome, *Psychiatric Quarterly, 51,* 39–54.

Leonard, C. V. (1973). What helps most about hospitalization? *Comprehensive Psychiatry, 14,* 365–369.

Moos, R., & Houts, P. (1968). Assessment of the social atmosphere of a psychiatric ward. *Journal of Abnormal Psychology, 73,* 595–604.

Murphey, S. A. (1979). Patients' and staff's perceptions of therapy in a short-term private psychiatric hospital. *International Journal of Nursing Studies, 16,* 159–167.

Pine, F., & Levinson, D. J. (1967). A sociopsychological conception of patienthood. *International Journal of Social Psychiatry, 71,* 106–121.

Small, I. F., Messina, J. A., & Small, J. G. (1964). The meaning of hospitalization: A comparison of attitudes of medical and psychiatric patients. *Journal of Nervous and Mental Disease, 13,* 575–579.

Small, I. F., Small, J. G., & Gonzales, R. (1965). The clinical correlates of attitudinal change during psychiatric treatment. *American Journal of Psychotherapy, 19,* 66–74.

Smith, H. L., & Thrasher, J. (1963). Roles, cliques and sanctions: Dimensions of patient society. *International Journal of Social Psychiatry, 9,* 184–191.

Soulem, O. (1955). Mental patients' attitudes towards mental hospitals. *Journal of Clinical Psychology, 11,* 181–185.

Stanton, A. H., & Schwartz, M. S. (1954). *The Mental Hospital.* New York: Basic Books.

Zaslove, M. C., Ungerleider, J. T., & Fuller, M. C. (1966). How psychiatric hospitalization helps: Patient views versus staff views. *Journal of Nervous and Mental Disease, 142,* 568–579.

<table>
<tr><td rowspan="2">4</td><td>

Depression and the Physically Ill
</td></tr>
<tr><td>

Priscilla Lynch
Marietta Nolan Stevens
</td></tr>
</table>

The identification of depression among the physically ill is underestimated and often overlooked. While depression is considered a normal response to illness, awareness of symptomatology indicating a major affective disorder becomes essential for accurate nursing assessment and intervention. This chapter describes theories of depression among the physically ill and provides the nurse with criteria for assessment as well as strategies for intervention.

REVIEW OF THE LITERATURE

Extent of the Problem

In contrast to the rate of depression in the general population, estimated to be from 4.5–8% (U.S. Department of Health and Human Services, 1980), the depression rate among the physically ill is higher than that found in the general population. The only studies that have looked at depression in the physically ill, or those adults with a physical or medical illness in addition to a clinical depression, found a range of 18–36%. While Moffic and Paykel (1975) discovered a rate of 24%, Cavanaugh (1983) found 36% of 335 medical patients to be depressed. In research conducted by Neilsen and Williams (1980), in which they examined the level of depression using the Beck Depression Inventory (BDI), they found 12.2% of 526 medical outpatients with mild depression, 5.5% with moderate depression, and 0.6% with severe depression.

NURSING INTERVENTIONS IN DEPRESSION   Copyright © 1985 by Grune & Stratton, Inc.
ISBN 0-8089-1710-2   All rights of reproduction in any form reserved.

Although a high rate of depression exists in the physically ill, it is often unrecognized by medical residents. According to Cavanaugh (1983), mild depression among the medically ill is not recognized 78% of the time; even more startling is that moderate to severe depression is undiagnosed 67% of the time. One reason that medical residents fail to recognize this condition is because its symptoms, such as anorexia or insomnia, also appear in other illnesses (Cavanaugh, et al., 1983).

A careful assessment of medical patients is suggested to avoid overlooking the symptoms of a clinical depression. Individuals showing signs of depressed mood or a slow recovery from illness may be harboring a depression. When the problem has been identified, a treatment plan should be initiated, focusing on the biological, psychological, and social needs of the depressed person.

Theories of Depression

The etiology of depression has long been an enigma for medical science. In "Mourning and Melancholia" (1957), Freud describes a syndrome of melancholia or depression after the loss of a loved one or object. Depressed persons feel unworthy and dissatisfied with themselves, ultimately resulting in loss of self-esteem.

Several other theories are advanced about the origin of depression. For example, social learning theory views depression as a learned behavior reinforced by other people or the environment. In a system's approach to depression, the depressed person is viewed as a dynamic system influenced by and influencing other systems, especially family and society (Marmor, 1983). With cognitive theorists, the depressed person's negative patterns of thought appear as the critical element of depression. It is conjectured that the thought patterns can be changed by cognitive restructuring (Beck, 1976).

In recent times, biochemical theories of depression have received increased attention in psychiatric circles. Depression may be related biochemically to the decrease of certain neurotransmitters at the synaptic receptor sites of the brain, such as norepinephrine and serotonin. Antidepressant drugs or electroshock therapy (ECT) may improve depression by correcting the imbalance of the biochemicals in the brain.

Depression has also been linked to an imbalance of the neuroendocrine system concerning the pituitary–adrenal feedback loop. Of clinical importance is the dexamethasone suppression test (DST) used to identify patients with endogenous depression. While normal subjects would suppress cortisol production, 50% of depressed patients fail to suppress cortisol output from the adrenal glands when given dexamethasone (a form of cortisol). The DST has been proven to be one of the few clinical indicators of depression.

The etiology of depression in the medically ill population may be more complex and interrelated. Depression has been found to precede, accompany, or follow a physical illness (Schwab, 1970). Depression may be the first symptom of certain diseases such as cancer or multiple sclerosis (Whitlock & Siskind, 1979; 1980); it can also accompany an acute illness such as a gastrointestinal or cardiovascular disorder (Schwab, et al., 1967; Kimball, 1977); or it can follow the illness in the recovery or rehabilitation period for patients with stroke, post-myocardial infarction, and chronic pain (Feibel & Springer, 1982; Magni & Bertolini, 1983; Taylor, et al., 1981). Often a question posed as to whether the depression is a reaction to the physical illness, or whether it is caused biologically by the physical illness itself (Whitlock, 1982). It is possible that the physical illness may deplete biochemicals in the brain. In such illnesses as multiple sclerosis, perhaps the plaques affect the levels of neurotransmitters in the brain to produce depression. It has also been suggested that patients in chronic pain may become depressed due to biological changes in neurotransmitters or neural pathways (Lindsay & Wyckoff, 1981).

Certain medications are known to create a depressive reaction in patients. The most well-known of these drugs, the antihypertensive reserpine, depletes stores of norepinephrine at the nerve endings, providing a model for the catecholamine theory of depression. Other drugs associated with depressive reactions are other antihypertensives, oral contraceptives, corticosteroids, anticancer drugs, and antiparkinson drugs (Klerman, 1981). Removal of the drug may improve the depression or antidepressants may be required. It is crucial to make a complete assessment of the patient's drug regime to prevent this problem.

Several researchers have examined the possible relationship of depression and cancer. One large longitudinal study concluded that depressed patients had a two-fold rate of death from cancer (Shekelle, et al., 1981). Other researchers have proposed the theory that depression may impair the individual's immune system, thus making him more susceptible to the spread of malignant cells (Kronfol, et al., 1983; Shekelle, et al., 1981; Whitlock & Siskind, 1979).

In addition to considering the biological component of depression, the psychological impact of a physical illness must be considered. Moos (1977) describes a physical illness as a life crisis, that of testing one's ability to cope or adapt. After the first shock of an acute illness, a normal period of depression follows in which the individual grieves loss of health or the ability to function as previously. During this time the person may feel sad and withdraw from others more than before until he or she can accept the condition or acknowledge the loss (Shontz, 1975). If the person is unable to acknowledge the illness and continues to withdraw for an extended period, a major depression may be diagnosed. According to the Diagnostic Statistical Manual of Mental Disorders (DSM-III) (American Psychiatric Association, 1980) a depression can result from the psychological reaction to a physical illness. Such a depression must be present with symptoms each day for at least 2 weeks. It is distinct from bereavement, a time-limited state of grief or depression that follows a death of a loved one.

In the person with a chronic illness, there are also adjustments in the process of accepting the illness. Straus (1975) discusses the life-style changes necessary to live with a chronic illness or disability. A chronically ill individual may slowly become more socially isolated and depressed. One study found symptoms of despair and hopelessness to be common in patients in the rehabilitation setting. If the rehabilitation is successful, these symptoms may abate, but if patients are unable to accept the chronic illness, it may lead to depression (Gans, 1981).

Depression may result from a biological change secondary to the physical illness itself, or may reflect a maladaptive response or inability to cope with the illness. In summary, considerably more data are needed to fully understand the etiology of depression in the physically ill.

NURSING ASSESSMENT

Symptomatology

The nurse working in the medical setting often encounters a patient who describes feeling "blue" or "sad." When this occurs the nurse must consider doing a psychological assessment of the patient. This assessment includes sitting down and talking with the patient about what he or she is experiencing. By encouraging the patient to describe feelings, the nurse can receive pertinent data from which to formulate an assessment. This assessment includes information not only from the patient but from significant others as well. Areas included in the psychological assessment are patient history, symptoms the patient describes, and the manner or behavior of the patient that nurse and significant others observe.

According to DSM-III criteria, a major affective disorder occurs when an individual experiences four of the following eight symptoms for a period of 2 weeks or longer. These symptoms include

1. Poor appetite or significant weight loss or increased appetite or significant weight gain.
2. Insomnia or hypersomnia.
3. Psychomotor agitation or retardation.
4. Loss of pleasure or interest in usual activities (anhedonia).
5. Loss of energy; fatigue.
6. Feelings of worthlessness or guilt.
7. Diminished ability to concentrate.
8. Recurrent thoughts of death or suicidal ideation (American Psychiatric Association, 1980)

However, for the medically ill individual the picture clouds and diagnosis is more difficult. Some of the symptoms of depression can be similar to those of physical illness and it becomes very important to consider all the interrelated factors affecting the individual.

The nurse begins a depression assessment by asking if there is any family history of depression or whether the individual has experienced depression before or since the onset of illness. Nurses can also question if the person is considering suicide or has attempted such in the past. If a positive response is verbalized, a further-detailed suicide assessment needs to be completed.

Questions related to the person's ability to experience pleasure and interest in activities may be addressed. Sample questions might be, "As a result of being ill, what activities have you stopped enjoying?" "If you were feeling better, how would it change?" "Do you find a difference in your ability to be interested in things?"

Feelings of hopelessness, helplessness, and loss of self-esteem can be indicative of depression as well. Patients may verbalize these feelings in ways such as, "Things will never improve," "I have nothing to look forward to," "I must have done something wrong," or "Who would want to listen to me?"

Loss of appetite and problems associated with sleep are factors that may indicate depression. Nurses need to be aware that these symptoms can be relative to the illness.

Differentiating symptoms of illness from symptoms of depression can be accomplished by assessing behavior patterns over a period of time. For example, if the patient has little or no appetite along with other depressive symptoms, even as the illness improves, this can be a indication that depression may be present. A continuing pattern of early morning awakenings or insomnia can be another indication of depression.

To accurately assess a patient's mood certain questions might be useful such as, "Can you describe how you are feeling right now?" "Would you describe your mood as being sad or blue?" "Do you find yourself crying more than usual?" Clark et al., (1983) document crying as a symptom discriminator for severity of depression especially in medical patients, whether or not they are able to explain why they are crying.

Additional assessment includes the nurse's observations of the patient's mood, affect, activity level, and environment. The patient's mood may have changed or been stable over time. When the patient verbalizes, there may be emotion communicated in facial expressions or voice tones. Check to see if the emotion is appropriate to the patient's verbalizations. Depressed patients often exhibit a flat nonemotional expression and voice tone or look sad. Body movements may be slowed with psychomotor retardation as well. Check to see if the patient's drapes drawn all the time or if the patient frequently stares off in to space or takes time to answer questions.

The patient's ability to concentrate can be useful in assessing depression. See if the patient is able to read and comprehend what he or she has read, or if the patient frequently cannot concentrate on specific tasks or projects.

Somatic complaints are frequently communicated by depressed patients. These complaints can be difficult to distinguish because they may be related to the physical illness as well. An increasing frequency of somatic complaints with other symptoms of depression present may provide a clue that depression is present. Although it is more difficult to identify symptoms of depression in the medically ill, the behaviors described will assist the nurse in identifying the depressed medical patient.

Assessing the Crisis State

In addition to the depression, the physically ill person may also be in a crisis state. For nurses, an individual perceived to be in crisis needs assessment, monitoring, and intervention. As defined by Caplan (1961), crisis occurs:

> when a person faces an obstacle to important life goals that is, for a time, insurmountable through the customary methods of problem solving. A period of disorganization ensues a period of upset during which many abortive attempts at solutions are made (Caplan, 1961).

Crisis also can be viewed as any rapid change or experience foreign to a person's usual experience (Hansell, 1976). Nevertheless, an unusual event happening to an individual does not necessarily mean a crisis state. According to Barrell, crisis is an "individual matter" (Barrell, 1974). Two people may experience the same situation, yet one will end up in crisis whereas the other will not. What then determines a crisis state?

The Aguilera and Messick model (1982) identifies three balancing factors to consider when assessing an individual for a crisis state: (1) realistic perception of the events; (2) situational supports; and (3) the individual's coping mechanisms. A crisis will not occur with all these factors in equilibrium, but when one becomes upset, a period of disequilibrium or a state of crisis results. It then becomes important during the assessment process to individually assess each of these three areas and look for a possible breakdown of the balancing factors resulting in a crisis situation.

As practitioners, nurses are familiar with the stress brought on by a physical illness. It is then easy to assume that the crisis is due to the illness or the accompanying hospitalizations, but that observation may be inaccurate. A patient brings along a repertoire of behaviors and problems that continue to be of concern while he or she is sick and hospitalized. Quite possibly a hospitalized individual may be in crisis because of an outside stress or event totally unrelated to the illness; or an individual may be experiencing a maturational or developmental crisis considered to be a normal and anticipated part of life. Some examples of developmental or maturational crises include role changes, puberty, and mid-life issues. Maturational or developmental crises usually occur around transition states as the individual moves from one developmental stage to another.

A situational or unanticipated crisis is one in which the individual has no control, such as developing a physical illness or becoming a patient in a hospital. One usually cannot prepare for this crisis. Assessment of the individual is necessary to determine the cause of the crisis—a developmental task, an unanticipated event or occurrence, or a combination of both.

It would be impossible for a person to remain in a crisis situation indefinitely (Hoff, 1984). Hoff identifies three possible outcomes of crisis (1) a return to the pre-crisis level of functioning; (2) a return not only to the pre-crisis state but a situation in which the individual actually grows from the experience; (3) or the individual decreases the intolerable tension by developing neurotic or psychotic behavior patterns, such as depression, withdrawal, or even suicide.

Assessing Suicidal Risk in a Medical Setting

Fawcett (1974) postulates that suicide is "an act that stems from some type of depression." If an individual is not depressed he will not commit suicide. That concept is an important one to keep in mind when assessing the suicidal individual.

Suicidal ideation may be present when the individual comes into the hospital as a patient. More commonly, suicidal behavior develops after the patient's medical condition is diagnosed or after he has been a patient in the hospital for a period of time. Suicidal thoughts or behaviors are a result of a depressive syndrome that may take the form of biochemical depression, reactive depression, or depression related to physical illness (Fawcett, 1974).

It is possible to identify persons with a higher suicide risk by assessing clinical variables, such as those who have attempted suicide before and people who have experienced the loss of very important persons in their life. This includes loss of parents early in life, loss of a spouse, a job, or a social role. It is important to keep in mind that threat of a loss can have as much impact as the real loss itself. Other clinical variables include people who are presently experiencing a depression or who are recovering from a depression, people who have a physical illness, especially when as a result of the illness there are body image changes, or the individual must make a life-style change. The final clinical variable is alcohol and substance abuse that results in decreased impulse control (Wilson & Kneisel, 1983).

There is a difference between a suicide attempt and a suicidal gesture. An attempt is defined as an act that would have resulted in an individual's death if there was no intervention of factors beyond the individual's control. A suicidal gesture is an act that may be viewed as being symbolic to suicide but of no serious threat to the individual (Bunney & Fawcett, 1968).

More often people who are suicidal will give cues regarding their intent. These cues can be of a verbal or nonverbal nature. A patient may verbally communicate a wish to die. Most often the response will be communicated indirectly with such responses as "I don't think I can go on much longer;" "What do I have to live for;" "What's the use of going on;" "Will you miss me when I'm gone?" An indirect way of expressing suicidal thoughts is in such nonverbal behaviors as changing or making out a will, giving away special possessions, becoming withdrawn, experiencing insomnia, and loss of interest in activities that were at one time very important to them. These are examples of behaviors that help us to recognize an individual who may become actively suicidal and attempt suicide while in the hospital setting.

A lethality assessment is also necessary to predict how likely the patient is to commit suicide. Once again, direct and open communication between patient and practitioner is necessary in order to complete this assessment. According to Fawcett (1974) and Hoff (1984), a lethality assessment includes a history of suicidal behavior or suicidal attempts. Included here are such factors as the method used, history of suicide in the family, and the outcome of the previous attempt. Another lethality factor is whether or not the individual has a suicide plan in mind and, if so, what means are they thinking of using. If the patient does speak of feeling suicidal, it becomes tantamount to assess whether the feelings are active (acute) or passive (subacute) nature. An active suicidal thought includes what the patient would like to accomplish with a specific plan for carrying out the wish. A passive suicidal thought is communicated in more vague terms with references to not wanting to be around or wishing to disappear (Fawcett, 1974).

The nurse must also question the patient about ways or methods used to commit suicide. Guns, knives, drowning, hanging, and certain groups of pills are considered high lethality methods. Cutting of the wrists and nonprescription drugs are usually considered low lethality methods.

In addition to assessing the lethality of the method, one must also consider if the method is available to the patient while he or she is in the hospital; e.g., if you are assessing a patient who plans to commit suicide by using sleeping pills, it becomes important to know whether or not the patient has the pills in the hospital. After doing a lethality and availability assessment, one also must question the patient as to the time and place the suicidal act will occur.

Thus when working with the medically ill patient who is suspected of being suicidal, one must consider if the patient is feeling depressed and hopeless. Is there a change in the patient's interactions with others—is he or she more withdrawn, regressed? Are there indicators that the individual is suicidal? All these factors provide clues to nurses caring for the medically ill patient.

NURSING INTERVENTION

Crisis and Suicide

According to the Aguilera and Messick (1982) model of crisis theory, the assessment process becomes the most important aspect of crisis intervention. Although the nurse's objectivity is essential, sometimes it becomes too difficult to curb feelings when working with patients. An example occurred with a 17-year old youth undergoing a bone marrow transplant. The patient's medical condition appeared stable. Suddenly the young man became anxious, withdrawn, and experienced insomnia. The health care team suspected this young man was in crisis although no one knew why. People suspected it was related to fears of dying. Finally the young man was able to verbalize that his girlfriend wanted to break up with him. Obviously, the crisis was not directly related to his being in the hospital or to his medical condition. Thus talking with the patient and obtaining the facts from his perspective was the first step in the intervention process.

The nurse plays an active role with the patient by guiding and directing the individual to solve the problem. The intervention plan must be developed collaboratively with the patient and significant others. Collaboration is important because if the patient does not have a vested interest in the plan, not much of a chance exists for the intervention to be successful.

Caplan and Grunebaum (1967) identify additional considerations in formulating an effective crisis intervention plan. As mentioned before, the plan focuses on the immediate problem that is directly responsible for the crisis.

The plan needs to be congruent with the individual's functional level and dependency needs. In other words, the more anxious a patient feels, the more active a role the nurse plays. Nurses need to accurately assess the dependence or independence of the patient that determines how active a role the nurse must assume. The therapeutic plan must be sensitive to the patient's life style and value system. Nurses must always keep in mind that various cultural, religious, and ethnic groups have individual responses to events of life, including physical illness. Crisis intervention plans must be realistic and concrete, so that a reassuring structure is provided for the individual patient. Intervention plans also need to be dynamic and renegotiable. If one plan does not work, a new one can be negotiated between the patient and nurse.

It is not at all unusual for the individual experiencing a crisis to be confused about the cause of the feelings of anxiety and unsettledness. The nurse assists by using such techniques as listening actively, encouraging the expression of feelings, helping the patient gain an understanding of the crisis and accept reality, and exploring new means of coping with problems (Hoff, 1984).

As nurses interact with patients experiencing a crisis, the goal is to also help them develop new and more effective coping behaviors for dealing with any problems they may experience throughout life. Anticipatory guidance or planning will also help patients to problem solve before an actual or anticipated problem becomes a reality. Patients experiencing a crisis in the hospital may find other issues in their life that need resolving. As a result, they express a desire to continue with therapy after leaving the hospital. Since this request is realistic, arrangements should be made to provide patients with a network prior to leaving the hospital.

One possible outcome of an unresolved crisis is the patient becoming actively suicidal. The nurse working with such a patient must give top priority to providing a safe environment. Since a medical milieu does not offer the same precautions provided on a psychiatric unit, several steps will need to be taken.

Suicide intervention on a medical floor calls for the removal of items considered hazardous such as firearms, knives, lighters and lighter fluid, matches, aerosol cans, and belts. Also included are belts to robes, shavers—both electric and straight edge,—medications, nail-polish remover, can openers, glass objects, and any sharp instruments. Routine safety checks may be necessary and, in addition, patients should be supervised when using any of the personal hygiene items considered dangerous.

One-to-one nursing observation should be required on a 24-hour basis as long as the patient remains actively suicidal. Corresponding documentation of the patient's status should be completed at least once every shift. Whenever possible medications in a liquid or injectible form are recommended. Mouth checks on the patient after receiving oral medication will assure the nurse that it has been swallowed.

The suicidal patient should be housed in a private room as close to the nurse station as possible and be restricted to the unit, leaving it only for diagnostic or therapeutic procedure.

A psychiatric consult is recommended as quickly as possible so that the psychiatrist can perform a psychiatric evaluation. Antidepressant and/or other psychotropic medication may be initiated.

Medical nurses often feel uncomfortable, anxious, and, overwhelmed with a suicidal patient on the unit. The psychiatric liaison nurse can be utilized effectively not only in conjunction with the suicidal patient but especially in providing support and expertise to medical nurses. The entire team working with suicidal patients aims to provide safety and comfort. If a psychiatric unit is available, it may be useful to consider transferring patients, if their condition warrants it.

Structuring the Environment For the Depressed Patient

In addition to intervening with the suicidal patient, another technique often helpful with depressed patients is structuring the environment. To structure means to form, build, or organize the elements. The nurse is an organizer and builder of the patient's environment, and shapes interactions between people and the schedule of the day's events. The goal becomes a calm, accepting, safe atmosphere where it is possible for the patient to recover a sense of hope and self-esteem (Mereness & Taylor, 1974).

Nursing looks at the biological, psychological, and social needs of the patient. Although nursing takes an interpersonal approach, focusing on the nurse–patient relationship, learning theories have shown that reinforcement is a powerful tool for creating observable behavior changes and thus relief of symptoms.

Wolf's (1977) review of the literature on milieu therapy reveals that the most successful programs are those that include order, organization, patient involvement, and a reasonable amount of staff control. Given these important elements, a nursing care plan for the depressed, physically ill person should include structured activities as well as considering psychological, social, and biological needs.

The need for structuring activities is apparent in the case of the depressed patient. The patient may describe a feeling of emptiness and disinterest, demonstrating a lack of desire to engage in activities. When the physically ill person becomes depressed, immediate and intensive assistance is needed; as the patient improves, and motivation and interest return, the need for such intervention is lessened.

By improving the structure of the patient's daily activities, and assisting the depressed patient in writing a schedule for the day, the nurse can provide boundaries for the patient, which often result in the patient's acquiring a sense of purpose. Activities such as exercise, physical therapy, or walks are helpful in providing for fitness and avoiding the complications of immobility. In addition, recent research has focused on relief of depression using physical exercise by possibly altering biochemicals in the brain (Ransford, 1982).

Occupational therapy or art therapy is available in most hospitals so that patients can work on projects that foster creativity and a sense of accomplishment. Other types of activities may also be available to give the patient opportunities to interact with other people. In the beginning of the depression, the patient may need strong encouragement to attend activities, but as the person becomes less depressed he or she will be more able to make his own choices.

Psychological Needs

Support can be viewed as that which strengthens the individual's ability to function competently at his or her level of satisfaction. It means helping someone carry on in the face of a difficult task requiring work. It does not mean that the person providing the support accomplishes the difficult task. Rather it aims to help the individual maintain personal wholeness by using his or her own internal resources in problem solving to accomplish the difficult task. Support as defined in this context really means emotional support.

Peplau (1952) views the nurse–patient relationship as a positive and helping one in which the patient can learn to trust another individual and to work through his various problems. When the same nurses work with patients on a daily basis a trust relationship can develop and the nurse serves as a source of emotional support. One of the most important factors to consider when providing emotional support to depressed individuals is to understand the needs of the patients as they describe them. The support giver provides empathic understanding of what the patient experiences. Providing patients with support communicates that someone cares about them, and this results in an increase in the individual's feelings of worth and self-esteem.

As an ongoing process, emotional support requires a commitment on the part of the care giver. A trusting relationship ensures that the patient will rely on the individual support giver, with the expectation that the relationship will provide a forum for that patient to identify feelings and needs and begin to problem solve in a healthy manner.

Nurses often show reluctance to provide emotional support for patients because they believe they lack the appropriate skills or techniques to be effective. Of greater concern, however, is the nurses' fear of saying the wrong thing or not knowing what to say in the face of a difficult or emotional interaction with the patient.

The psychological needs of the depressed person on a medical unit may be overlooked because of the time necessary to care for other patients with more pressing conditions. Nurses caring for depressed, physically ill individuals must plan their time to allow for sufficient time for interactions with patients. One approach might be for the nurse to meet with a patient at a prearranged time during the shift. In this way the patient is insured the opportunity to verbalize his or her feelings about the illness and other concerns.

The following case illustrates this approach.

Mr. A., a 74-year-old man with lung cancer was hospitalized on a medical unit where he soon became depressed. He neither spoke nor showed any interest in eating. He progressively lost weight, becoming too weak to leave his bed. His nurses developed a plan that included half-hour sessions with Mr. A. in his room each morning and evening. During those periods, the nurses focused primarily on the patient's psychological needs. The nurses did not force a response from Mr. A. but sat with him in his room. When a nurse was not with him the door to his room was left open, so that he could observe people walking by. After a few days, the patient began to speak about his fear of death. He also expressed his grief concerning his wife's death, and also began to eat slowly and regained more strength. The attention to Mr. A.'s psychological needs arrested his increasing withdrawal.

Safety and security is another psychological need that nurses must provide. A sense of security and safety is crucial to the therapeutic environment fostered by consistent communication and limit-setting by the nursing staff (Holmes & Werner, 1966). To maintain a secure environment, inappropriate or unsafe behavior would be dealt with at the time it occurs.

Mary's case represents the importance of limit setting. Although she denied bringing medication to the hospital, Mary was observed taking a valium from her purse. When queried the patient said: They wouldn't give me enough to relax me. I wanted to have my own pills just in case.'' In this instance, Mary's nurse explained to her that patients taking their own medication to the hospital could not be monitored and the practice was therefore not permitted. The pills were taken away from Mary, but returned to her at the time of discharge, at which time advice in the proper use of medication was given.

Helping to meet the psychological needs of the patient is not the only method for treating the depressed medical patient, but when utilized in conjunction with other nursing interventions it can be of extreme benefit to the individual patient.

Social Needs

The depressed patient often experiences impaired interpersonal relationships resulting in isolative behavior. Strategies that nurses can use in decreasing this isolation include placing the patient in a room with an appropriate roommate, encouraging family to visit, and providing opportunities for the patient to be out of his or her room, such as touring the hospital accompanied by a volunteer or family member.

Opportunities for socialization may be available on the medical unit. Discussion groups directed by psychiatric clinical specialists need to focus on the communication processes of listening, responding, and providing support to others. Some patients frequently discover that others have similar feelings or experiences related to illness and depression. Thus, in the group, they learn to share coping strategies with each other. It may be beneficial to involve patients with talking about the impact of the patient's illness.

Biological Needs

As in Mr. A.'s case, medical problems of depressed patients, such as anorexia and weight loss, unquestionably exacerbate existing physical problems. Therefore, nurses must be alerted to potential complications.

In situations in which anorexia occurs, the nurse can talk with the patient about food likes and dislikes in order to obtain desirable meals. Since patients often say they are "too full to eat anymore," an appropriate tactic could be to offer snacks and juices in between meals. Food and fluid intake and daily weight should be monitored to avoid further weight loss, dehydration, or electrolyte imbalances. It may be helpful to tell patients that, while they may not have an appetite for food at the time, their appetite will improve as the depression abates.

Such sleep disturbances as insomnia, early morning awakenings, or interrupted sleep, appear frequently in depression. With the use of relaxation techniques that focus on decreasing muscle tension, nurses can teach patients to relax before bedtime. Depressed patients often fixate on their sleeping problems and spend the day trying to nap to "make-up" the missed sleep. The nurse can point out that sleep will improve with antidepressant medication. Also, naps do not help to restore sleep patterns.

Constipation appears to be a common problem in the depressed patients who has minimal physical exercise and a poor diet, and it is also a side effect of antidepressant medication. The nurse will need to monitor bowel function because many patients ignore this area until a problem occurs. Instructions in diet, hydration, and exercise should be given.

Fostering More Adaptive Coping

Coping is a process in which the person seeks to maintain a psychological balance to meet an environmental challenge, to decrease pain and suffering, to obtain new information, or to increase competence (Hamburg, et al., 1974). For coping to be successful, one must be "flexible, rational, and effective" in problem solving (Lazarus, et al., 1974). A person who is depressed often feels restricted in the alternatives available for coping with various situations (Arieti & Bemporad, 1980). The nurse in such situations can help the patient consider alternatives. Note the following example:

Mr. G. became depressed after a myocardial infarction and bypass surgery. He refused to leave his apartment, fearing that he would have a heart attack if he went outside or to the store. After several trips to the emergency room for chest pains, during which all tests were normal, Mr. G. was hospitalized. Although the nursing care plan considered his physical condition, it focused on his depression and isolative behavior. With the help of his primary nurse, Mr. G. agreed to formulate one new goal for each day to lessen his anxiety. He became interested in leather crafts in occupational therapy, receiving complements from patients and staff on his work. His self-confidence increased to the point where he attended a discussion group in which he found support among other patients, and he gradually became involved in more social situations and was more verbal about his opinions. In daily conferences with his primary and associate nurses, he discussed his fears since his heart attack, as well as his reluctance to be around people or to try new activities. Next, with the cardiologist's approval, Mr. G. started a walking program. First accompanied by a staff member, he later ventured alone outside the hospital. Upon accomplishing each new goal, his attitude and mood improved. After discharge, the patient agreed to participate in social events at the senior citizens center and continue his walking. Through alternative strategies, Mr. G. became more self sufficient.

When a patient can choose goals and strategies, he may feel more responsible for and in control of his own treatment.

R., a security guard on disability leave from work because of chronic back pain, became so dependent on prescribed narcotics, that hospitalization was required. Pale and frowning, he would often tell the nurses that they didn't understand how much pain he endured. To show his disapproval that the pain medication was not scheduled more frequently, he frequently came to the nurses' station saying "Can't I have something now? I take a lot stronger medication at home." He became angry if the medication was not yet scheduled. R.'s nurse talked to the patient about his behavior regarding the medication schedule, and allowed him to vent his feelings. He complained, "Those nurses are just trying to control me by not giving me enough medication for the pain." R., his nurse, and the doctor discussed the goal of managing R.'s pain with non-narcotic drugs, working out a schedule in which the medication would be given more frequently upon R's request. R.'s behavior improved and he reported the pain was more manageable after he gave input into the treatment plan.

In some situations, the family becomes too involved with the patient allowing the person to remain in the "sick role."

Mr. W., a 60-year-old man with Parkinson's disease had become increasingly depressed at home. As the disease progressed and walking became more difficult, he would demand that his family stay with him. In the hospital the family hovered over Mr. W. most of the day, making requests of the nursing staff on his behalf.

The treatment approach included adjusting the medication for the Parkinson's disease so that he could move more freely. As a result, he was able to walk with a cane, although he was reluctant to leave his bed or talk to any other patients. After establishing a relationship with his primary and associate nurses, the patient was more willing to dress and to come out of his room. The nurses kept in close contact with the family, educating them about the symptoms of depression and about Parkinson's disease. The family was urged to limit the time they came to visit the patient so he could be more self-reliant. Slowly, Mr. W. did more things for himself and the family was less anxious about caring for him, freeing Mr. W. from his "sick role."

In summary, the nurse can assist the patient in developing more adaptive coping by allowing him or her to consider a wide range of alternative behaviors. Strategies should encompass giving the patient choices in treatment, and helping the patient work towards self-generated goals. The patient and the family can benefit from the independence engendered by these adaptive coping approaches.

Psychiatric Consultation

Often, the depressed medical patient requires additional intervention, either from a psychiatric liaison nurse, a psychiatrist, or both.

The psychiatric liaison nurse is a master's-prepared clinical specialist. The psychiatric liaison nurse works directly with the patient, with staff only, or with both patient and staff. A liaison nurse may perform a psychiatric assessment on the patient and recommends a nursing care plan to the staff. Depressed patients often will respond to someone who visits with them on a regular basis and helps them to focus on their depressed feelings. When the nursing staff caring for these individuals experiences a sense of failure and frustration, the psychiatric liaison nurse can work directly with the staff to provide support and problem-solving strategies. Usually, better communication, which results in decreased feelings of failure on the part of the nursing staff, is the result of the intervention.

A psychiatrist may evaluate the patient to determine the type of depression and the possible response to antidepressant medication. The psychiatrist may determine that the patient requires a more structured environment, such as a psychiatric unit.

The psychiatric liaison nurse and the psychiatrist can work together caring for the same patient. A case conference on the patient provides a formalized mechanism in which all staff members working with the patient can share ideas, concerns, and problem solve to formulate a plan of care beneficial to the depressed patient. Including the individual patient in the conference whenever possible, makes the patient an active participant in the care plan. If the patient cannot participate in the conference, keeping him or her informed and up-to-date becomes a priority task for the health care team.

SUMMARY

As previously discussed, depression among the physically ill is more common than in the general population. First the patient needs to be assessed for symptoms of depression, crisis, and suicide. After the depressed physically ill patient is identified, nursing interventions include structuring of the environment, meeting psychological, social, and biological needs, and fostering adaptive coping.

Crisis situations, such as a suicidal patient, require immediate intervention on the part of the nursing staff. Utilizing psychiatric liaison nurses and/or psychiatrists can help the nursing staff provide appropriate care for the patient.

Knowledge of depression and new treatment modalities can be especially helpful to the nurse providing care for the depressed medically ill.

REFERENCES

American Psychiatric Association. (1980). *Diagnostic and statistical manual of mental disorders* (3rd ed.). Washington, D.C.: American Psychiatric Association.

Aguilera, D. & Messick, J. (1982). *Crisis intervention: Theory and methodology* (4th ed.). St. Louis: C. V. Mosby Company.

Arieti, S., & Bemporad, J. R. (1980). The psychological organization of depression. *American Journal of Psychiatry, 137*(11), 1360–1365.

Barrell, L. M. (1974). Crisis intervention—partnership in problem solving. *Nursing Clinics of North America, 9*(1), 5–17.

Beck, A. T. (1976). *Cognitive therapy and the emotional disorders*. New York: The New American Library, Inc.

Bunney, W. E., Jr., & Fawcett, J. (1968). Biochemical research in depression and suicide. *Suicidal behaviors: Diagnosis and management*. Boston: Little Brown and Company.

Caplan, G. (1961). *An approach to community mental health* (p. 18). New York: Grune & Stratton.

Caplan, G., & Grunebaum, H. (1967). Perspective on primary prevention, a review. *Archives of General Psychiatry, 17*(9), 331–346.

Cavanaugh, S. A. (1983). The prevalence of emotional and cognitive dysfunction in a general medical population: Using the MMSE, GHQ and BDI. *General Hospital Psychiatry, 5,* 15–24.

Cavanaugh, S., Clark, D. C., & Gibbons, R. T. (1983). Diagnosing depression in the hospitalized medically ill. *Psychosomatics, 24*(9), 809–815.

Clark, D. C., Cavanaugh, S. A., & Gibbons, R. D. (1983). The core symptoms of depression in medical and psychiatric patients. *Journal of Nervous and Mental Disease, 171*(12), 705–713.

Fawcett, J. (1974). Clinical assessment of suicidal risk. *Postgraduate medicine, 35*(3), 85–89.

Feibel, J. H., & Springer, C. J. (1982). Depression and failure to resume social activities after stroke. *Archives of Physical Medicine and Rehabilitation, 63,* 276–278.

Freud, S. (1957). Mourning and melancholia. In J. Strachey (Ed.), *The standard edition of the complete psychological works of Sigmund Freud* (Vol. 14) (pp. 243–258). London: The Hogarth Press.

Gans, J. S. (1981). Depression diagnosis in a rehabilitation hospital. *Archives of Physical Medicine and Rehabilitation, 62*(8), 386–389.

Hamburg, D. A., Coelho, G. V., & Adams, J. E. (1974). Coping and adaptation: Steps towards a synthesis of biological and social perspectives. In G. V. Coelho, D. A. Hamburg, & J. E. Adams (Eds.), *Coping and adaptation* (pp. 403–440). New York: Basic Books, Inc.

Hansell, N. (1976). *The person in distress.* New York: Human Service Press.

Hoff, L. (1984). *People in crisis: Understanding and helping.* Menlo Park: Addison-Wesley Publishing Co.

Holmes, M. J., & Werner, J. A. (1966). *Psychiatric nursing in a therapeutic community* (pp. 43–63). New York: MacMillan.

Kimball, C. P. (1977). Psychologic responses to the experience of open heart surgery. In R. Moos (Ed.), *Coping with physical illness* (pp. 113–133). New York: Plenum Medical Book Corporation.

Klerman, G. L. (1981). Depression in the medically ill. *Psychiatric Clinics of North America, 4*(2), 301–317.

Kronfol, Z., Silva, J., Jr., Greden, J., Dembinski, S., Gardiner, R., & Carroll, B. (1983). Impaired lymphocyte function in depressive illness. *Life Sciences, 33,* 241–247.

Lazarus, R. S., Averill, J. R., & Opton, E. M. (1974). The psychology of coping: Issues of research and assessment. In G. V. Coelho, D. A. Hamburg, and J. E. Adams (Eds.), *Coping and adaptation.* (pp. 249–315). New York: Basic Books, Inc.

Lindsay, P. G., & Wyckoff, M. (1981). The depression–pain syndrome and its response to antidepressants. *Psychosomatics, 22*(7), 571–577.

Magni, G., & Bertolini, C. (1983). Chronic pain as a depressive equivalent. *Postgraduate Medicine, 73*(3), 79–85.

Marmor, J. (1983). Systems thinking in psychiatry: Some theoretical and clinical implications. *American Journal of Psychiatry, 140*(7), 833–838.

Mereness, D. A., & Taylor, C. M. (1974). *The essentials of psychiatric nursing* (9th ed.). St. Louis: The C. V. Mosby Company.

Moffic, H. S., & Paykel, E. S. (1975). Depression in medical in-patients. *British Journal of Psychiatry, 126,* 346–353.

Moos, R. H. (1977). *Coping with physical illness.* New York: Plenum Medical Book Company.

Nielsen, A. C., & Williams, T. (1980). Depression in ambulatory medical patients. *Archives of General Psychiatry, 37,* 999–1004.

Peplau, H. (1952). *Interpersonal relations in nursing.* New York: G. P. Putnam's Sons.

Ransford, C. P. (1982). A role for amine in the antidepressant effect of exercise: A review. *Medicine and Science in Sports and Exercise,* 1982, *14*(1), 1–10.

Schwab, J. J. (1970). Depression in medical and surgical patients. In A. J. Enelow (Ed.), *Depression in medical practice.* West Point, Penn.: Merck & Company, Inc.

Schwab, J. J., Bialow, M., Brown, J. M., & Holzer, C. E. (1967). Diagnosing depression in medical inpatients. *Annals of Internal Medicine, 67*(4), 695–707.

Shekelle, R. B., Raynor, W. J., Ostfeld, A. M., Garron, D. C., Bieliauskas, L. A., Liu, S. C., Maliza, C., & Paul, O. (1981). Psychological depression and 17-year risk of death from cancer. *Psychosomatic Medicine, 43*(2), 117–125.

Shontz, F. C. (1975). *The psychological aspects of physical illness and disability.* New York: MacMillan Publishing Company.

Straus, A. L. (1975). *Chronic illness and the quality of life.* St. Louis: C. V. Mosby.

Taylor, C. B., DeBusk, R. F., Davidson, D. M., Houston, N., & Burnett, K. (1981). Optimal methods for identifying depression following hospitalization for myocardial infarction. *Journal of Chronic Diseases, 34*(4), 127–133.

U.S. Department of Health and Human Services. Public Health Service Alcohol, Drug Abuse, and Mental Health Administration. (1980). *The alcohol, drug abuse, and mental health national data book.* Rockville, Maryland: U.S. Department of Health and Human Services.

Whitlock, F. A. (1982). *Symptomatic affective disorders.* New York: Academic Press.

Whitlock, F. A., & Siskind, M. (1979). Depression and cancer: A follow-up study. *Psychological Medicine, 9,* 747–752.

Whitlock, F. A., & Siskind, M. M. (1980). Depression as a major symptom of multiple sclerosis. *Journal of Neurology, Neurosurgery, and Psychiatry, 43*(1), 861–865.

Wilson, H. S., & Kneisl, C. R. (1983). *Psychiatric nursing* (2nd ed.). Menlo Park: Addison-Wesley Publishing Company.

Wolf, M. S. (1977). A review of literature on milieu therapy. *Journal of Psychiatric Nursing and Mental Health Services, 15*(5), 26–33.

5	# Sleep and Depression ## Rosalind D. Cartwright

Anyone who has worked with depressed patients knows that they often experience severe sleep disturbances. Some sleep too much, most sleep too little. It is now possible to do more than list this as one of the diagnostic signs of affective disorder. Now the type of sleep disturbance specific to depression can be identified and, more importantly, can be used diagnostically to differentiate these patients from other psychiatric patients and from nondepressed poor sleepers. It can also be used prognostically to predict treatment response. Further, recognition of this sleep profile has been used to develop new experimental treatments for depression designed to correct sleep disorders directly, rather than indirectly through the use of pharmacological agents. This work has led to new theoretic models of underlying biological disorders that gives rise to both the sleep and waking depressive symptoms. All of these gains have taken place over the past dozen years through a major effort to understand sleep troubles of the depressed. This effort is still yielding new insights into the nature of depression. As a result, this area of study is of major interest to those in pyschiatric nursing who are in a position to observe the patient throughout the 24-hour cycle and who care for patients during their troubled sleep.

HISTORY OF MODERN SLEEP AND DREAM RESEARCH

When the modern era of sleep and dream research opened in the mid 1950s (Aserinsky & Kleitman, 1953; Dement & Kleitman, 1957), with the more precise laboratory methods of approaching the study of the unconscious, there was an anticipation that this work might produce new insights in the area of mental illness. The first findings, that sleep is not homogeneous but consists of two distinct types—Rapid Eye Movement (REM) sleep and Nonrapid Eye Movement (NREM) sleep—and that each is associated with a distinct psychological activity, were soon followed by a series of other findings that changed the basic premises about mental life. REM sleep was so reliably associated with the experience of hallucinatory fantasies (dreams), and NREM with thought-like realistic cognition, that it was no longer tenable to think of the mind as turned off during sleep. Further, these two sleep states alternated so predictably across the night that dreaming could no longer be considered a sporadic occurrence. Any mental activity so frequent in all normal persons and predictable in its appearance must surely be serving some basic function.

To investigate what this dream function might be, experiments were conducted in which REM sleep was suppressed. The technique was crude but effective. The sleeper was awakened each time he or she was about to enter the REM stage. The effects of this manipulation were clear. REM deprivation was followed by an increase in REM percent on the first night of ad-lib sleep (Dement, 1960). The first REM period also appeared earlier in the night, as if the deprivation resulted in more pressure for this state. Even during experimental nights, while REM was being curtailed, the number of awakenings needed to prevent it tended to increase. The greater the restriction, the more REM attempts appeared in the electroencephalogram (EEG) record. These findings were interpreted as demonstrating that there is a need for dreaming and, further, that if dreaming were prevented from its normal cyclic appearance, it might come to intrude into waking life in the form of hallucinations. It was thought that perhaps REM deprivation might provide an experimental model of schizophrenia, but further work did not support this. None of the subjects developed psychotic symptoms during REM deprivation unless they were already bordering on a breakdown, and the early hope that the study of sleep might increase the understanding of this major mental disorder faded early.

Another decade passed before the field of mental illness was approached again through sleep studies. In this case, the area of affective disorders was examined. Here EEG of sleep revealed striking abnormalities. It seemed reasonable that there would be differences between the EEG recorded sleep of the depressed and normal sleep values on the basis of clinical reports of poor sleep and early morning awakenings in these patients. When these patients were monitored all night their sleep showed reduced amounts of delta sleep (EEG stages 3 and 4) and increases in arousals throughout the night. The findings were not specific to affective disorders; these indications of lighter and more disrupted sleep were also characteristic of the sleep of alcoholics and those with other major medical and psychiatric illnesses. However, these early studies had basic design flaws; e.g., the samples were often heterogeneous in diagnosis and in treatment status. Often medications were uncontrolled and the data analyses assumed all depressed persons were alike and lumped together inpatients, outpatients, neurotic, psychotic, endogenous, reactive, bipolar, and unipolar types.

At that time the field of differential psychiatric diagnosis was undergoing a period of rapid development to established standardized criteria (Feighner et al. 1972), and there was a parallel development in the field of sleep. The first standardized scoring procedures were adopted by Rechtschaffen and Kales (1968). These two standardized systems paved the way for better-controlled studies of the sleep of the depressed. The first sleep studies employing well-diagnosed patient groups reported those with primary depression had distinctive sleep characteristics and, what is more, these were identified as being specific to the REM sleep state.

Kupfer and his colleagues (Kupfer & Foster, 1972; 1976; Kupfer, et al., 1978) published a series of papers reporting that those with primary depression, i.e., with no previous psychiatric history, have a shortened interval before the appearance of the first REM sleep period of the night (i.e., REM latency). The identification of this distortion in the sleep architecture from that of normal controls was quickly confirmed in studies by Gillin et al., 1979; Duncan et al., 1979; G. Vogel et al., 1980; and Feinberg et al., 1982. All reported REM latency in hospitalized primary (endogenous) depressives to average about 45–50 minutes. This is just half the REM latency of normal age-matched subjects. Other studies extended this finding to different groups of depressed patients. Rush et al. (1982) reported outpatients to average 54 minutes. Bipolar, unipolar, and delusional patients, and patients with schizoaffective disorders all showed this sign in contrast to normals and to those with nonaffective psychiatric diagnoses.

In addition to REM latency, there were other REM parameters reported to be distorted in those with affective disorders. The distribution of REM sleep is often shifted from the normal proportion of one-third in the first half of the night and two-thirds in the second half, to a more equal distribution in the two halves—or even a more pronounced appearance in the first than the second half of the night (G. Vogel et al., 1980).

A third finding reported that the first REM period of the night in the depressed can be prolonged in comparison to that of normal control subjects (G. Vogel et al., 1980). A normal first REM averages 10–12 minutes, whereas in the depressed this may last 30 minutes or more. All of these observations relate to what are called the tonic, or continuous, elements of REM sleep. There are other differences that have been noted between the phasic elements of the REM sleep of depressive patients and normal controls. The first is an increase in REM density during the first REM period of the night. This is established by rating or counting the number of rapid eye movements in each minute of REM sleep divided by the number of minutes in that REM period. There is also an uneven distribution of these movements within REM periods; there can be periods of minutes of quiescence followed by eye-movement storms (Hauri & Hawkins, 1971). In addition, there may be an irregular sequence of REM density in the night's sleep. Instead of the usual increase in eye-movement density from beginning to end, the last REM period might have fewer eye movements per minute than the first (Cartwright, 1983). Thus, of the six disturbances listed, three are properties specific to the first REM:

1. This period occurs earlier in the night (half the normal latency).
2. It is often more prolonged in duration (twice the normal length).
3. It is often more active in terms of frequency of eye movements.

The other REM sleep distortions refer to the night as a whole:

4. The distribution of REM sleep tends to be shifted toward the first half of the night.
5. No-eye-movement intervals are followed by eye-movement storms.
6. The sequence of REM density measures across the night is frequently irregular.

DIFFERENTIAL DIAGNOSIS ON THE BASIS OF SLEEP STUDIES

Given this picture of a disturbance of both tonic and phasic REM features in the depressed, the next question is whether these features are unique to affective disorder and, if so, which are critical in discriminating these patients from other groups. A between-group strategy has been employed to answer these questions. A study by Gillin et al. (1979) compared the sleep of 56 hospitalized depressive patients to that of 41 normal volunteers and 18 primary insomnia patients. They used a univariate analysis in which pair-wise comparisons were made. When normals were compared to insomniacs, the normals had more total sleep, a shorter latency to sleep onset, more delta sleep, and a higher percentage of sleep-time (greater sleep efficiency) while in bed. When normals were compared to the depressed, normals again showed more total sleep, shorter latency to initial sleep, less early morning waking, more delta, greater sleep efficiency, and longer latency to the first REM period. When insomniacs were compared to the depressed, the latter showed more early morning awakening, shorter REM latency, and greater REM density. A discriminant analysis was performed using these sleep variables. This analysis succeeded in correctly classifying 100% of the normals, 73% of the depressed, and 78% of the insomniacs.

Using another strategy, groups within the broad category of affective disorders were compared. Reynolds et al. (1982) reported that 20 inpatients with a diagnosis of major affective illnesses differed from 20 age-matched outpatients in the degree of their REM sleep disturbance. Inpatients showed shorter REM sleep latencies and higher eye-movement density in the first REM. Thus, it appears the difference between these groups is one of severity. Coble et al.

(1976) also reported differences between two groups; one with a diagnosis of primary, the other of secondary depression. Again, the primary group had shorter REM latency, greater REM density, and more mixtures of Stage 2 and REM sleep. It appears that the sleep EEG is a useful diagnostic aid in separating the affective disorders from other diagnostic groups with poor sleep, and in estimating the degree of severity within depressive groups.

TREATMENT PROGNOSIS

Knowing the sleep characteristics associated with a major depression raises the question of response of these distortions to treatment. In earlier studies the assumption was that REM sleep markers were state variables that would return to normal values with remission of the depressive episode. Certainly shortened REM latency could be normalized within the first two nights following the introduction of antidepressant medication to those who responded well to this type of depression relief treatment. This is impressive since the change in waking clinical state might take as much as 3 weeks to become apparent. It is interesting that a REM latency criterion of 50 minutes or less can be used to predict response to amitriptyline (Svendsen & Christensen, 1981). In one study patients with normal or longer latencies to the first REM period were not only nonresponders to antidepressant medication, but were later diagnosed as falling into a neurotic depression rather than an endogenous diagnosis. In other words, an abnormally shortened latency to REM sleep is predictive of a positive response to this antidepressant medication probably because one action of this agent is to suppress REM sleep. This effect corrects the early REM distortion of sleep architecture and is in some fashion correlated to clinical improvement.

To test the hypothesis that the key to the therapeutic effectiveness of an antidepressant agent is that it prevents abnormal REM from occuring, several investigators have attempted to treat depressed patients by keeping them awake all night for one or two nights. This strategy has resulted in positive but transitory clinical effects. These studies, while disappointing as direct treatments, were supportive of the proposition that depressed patients feel better when the abnormal sleep pattern is prevented expression. The next step was taken by Wirz-Justice et al. (1976) who used clinical response following one night of sleep deprivation as a predictive indicator for the subsequent effectiveness of clomipramine versus maprotiline. Their findings, which have since been replicated by Fahndrich (1983), show a clear association: those patients responding positively to one night of total sleep deprivation did well with a serotonergic antidepressant, whereas those who did not were more likely to respond to a noradrenergic antidepressant agent. Thus, sleep deprivation appears to be a simple yet powerful aid in selecting the class of pharmacologic agents most likely to succeed. These associations still leave open the question of the relationship of specific REM sleep dysfunction to depressive symptoms. This has been addressed in another fashion in studies in which only the REM stage of sleep is restricted in order to test the effectiveness of REM sleep deprivation as a primary treatment rather than a prediction of response to subsequent drug treatment.

SLEEP TREATMENTS

The major study in this area was carried out by G. Vogel et al. (1975), who approached the question of whether therapeutic effectiveness of antidepressent agents was due to their REM-suppressing qualities by designing a study to test the effect of REM deprivation when used without medication on depressive patients. This landmark study included 34 patients with an endogenous diagnosis and 18 with a diagnosis of reactive depression. The deprivation of the REM stage of sleep was accomplished by monitoring the sleep of all patients in the laboratory, including the usual EEG, eye movement (EOG), and muscle tonus (EMG) parameters needed to identify REM sleep. When the sleep recording showed the REM stage had begun, the patient was awakened to abort that episode and kept awake for a few minutes to prevent the patient from immediately returning to REM sleep. This routine was carried out for 6 consecutive nights or until 30 awakenings per night were needed to prevent REM from occurring. Since, as was noted earlier, REM deprivation is followed by increased REM time and earlier REM attempts, and depressed persons already suffer from early REM onset, this routine might be expected to produce only temporary improvement followed by relapse when the restriction on REM sleep is lifted. Also, temporary effects produced in the studies of both 1 and 2 nights of sleep deprivation point to the need for longer periods of treatment. G. Vogel et al. (1975) worked out a way to extend the REM-suppressing treatment over several weeks by giving a night of ad-lib sleep whenever the number of awakenings criterion (six nights of REM deprivation or a night on which 30 awakings were needed to prevent REM) had been reached.

The study was carefully controlled using a double blind cross-over design. Half the group were in the REM-awakening experimental condition first while the other half had an equal number of NREM awakenings as a control condition. The experimental subjects were then crossed over into the control condition while the controls had the REM-suppressing experimental awakenings. All psychotropic medication was discontinued and patients remained drug-free during the study. By the conclusion of the study, 17 of the 34 endogenous patients had improved sufficiently to be discharged after 7 weeks of REM-suppression treatment. In other words, half of the patients did respond and half did not. Eleven of the failures were treated with imipramine, and 10 were unimproved on this medication. Seven of those who failed to respond to both treatments were given Electroconvulsive therapy (ECT), and 6 responded well enough to leave the hospital.

The story for the endogenous patients was straightforward. The half who improved with direct REM suppression would probably have improved on imipramine, and the half who failed to respond to the experimental treatment also failed to respond to this medication. It took a markedly different treatment (ECT) to be effective for REM-deprivation endogenous failures. ECT does not suppress REM sleep and so has a different course of action.

The story is quite different for the patients whose diagnosis was reactive depression. Although 13 of the 18 patients improved enough to leave the hospital, the improvement could not be attributed to REM deprivation. Controls who had only NREM awakenings improved at the same rate as experimentals during their exposure to the REM awakening routine. Vogel et al. (1975) concluded that REM deprivation is specific for the endogenous diagnosis, but that even this group is heterogeneous, containing two biologically distinct subgroups: REM-suppression responders and ECT responders.

A second study by G. Vogel et al. (1980), compared the effects of REM sleep deprivation on 14 endogenously depressed and 14 nondepressed insomnia patients using the same routine as in the first study. The additional insights provided by this study indicated that improvement in depression correlated with increased REM percent at the end of the night as well as with increased REM pressure on the recovery night (total REM percent increase over baseline). Vogel and associates concluded that the sleep problem in depression is that there is a failure to inhibit early REM so that Stages 3 and 4 can occur at the beginning of the night. The imposed experimental inhibition of REM acts to stimulate the "REM inhibitor" to function more efficiently. This hypothesis, of a disturbance in the timing of the REM cycle in affective disorder causing REM to be released earlier, is part of a new way of modeling this disorder and new ways of approaching its treatment.

THE PHASE ADVANCE HYPOTHESIS

It has been noted by several investigators that the sleep architecture of the depressed, with its characteristic earlier REM in the beginning of the night and early offset of sleep (early morning awakening), looks remarkably like the second half of a normal sleep cycle (Figures 5-1 and 5-2). This led to the hypothesis that depressives may suffer from a phase-advance of the REM sleep circadian rhythm (Kripke et. al., 1978). There is some support of this hypothesis from a comparative study of the temperature cycle of 10 bipolars and 14 normal controls (Wehr et al., 1980). The depressed showed an earlier low point of temperature in the night and earlier morning high-point than did normals. Another piece of evidence comes from comparing the sleep architecture of normal subjects, whose sleep onset time is delayed by several hours, to the architecture that is typical of

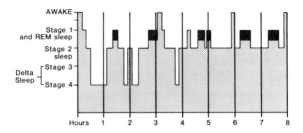

Fig. 5-1. Typical sleep pattern of a young human adult. Stage 1 sleep and REM sleep are graphed on the same level because their EEG patterns are very similar.

the depressed. Several studies (Taub & Berger, 1976; Webb et al., 1971; Weitzman et al., 1970) showed that under these circumstances the first REM period also occurred early, at about the same range of latencies (40–55 minutes) as is usually reported for the depressed. Delaying sleep onset seems to advance REM sleep propensity. Vogel et al. (1980) suggested that the REM phase advance in depressives might be the result of their chronically poor sleep.

This again raises the question: Is the REM sleep abnormality an effect or is it involved in the pathogenesis of the affective disorders? The evidence is not conclusive at this point, but there are scattered observations to support that the abnormally advanced REM cycle precedes rather than follows the clinical picture of depression. D. J. Kupfer (personal communication, 1980) has observed a

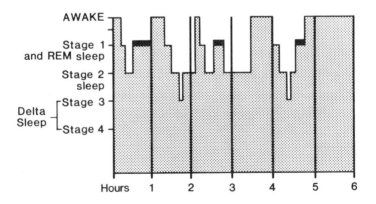

Fig. 5-2. Typical sleep pattern in depression.

profound shortening of REM latency in a patient on maintenance medication with a score on the Hamilton Scale of Depression (1967) of zero just before her clinical relapse. In rapidly cycling manic-depressive patients who have been studied longitudinally (Wehr et al., in press), REM latency has been shown to become progressively shorter during the manic phase until switching to depression, at which time this value progressively lengthens. This appears to support the theory that the REM latency cycle parallels but precedes the mood cycle.

To test these ideas Wehr et al. (1979) attempted to affect the mood of 6 bipolar patients by advancing their sleep time by 6 hours, thinking that perhaps this would allow the REM cycle to occur in a more normal relation to the sleep cycle. Three patients experienced total remission and 2 had partial remissions, and although these were temporary, they supported the idea that the phase advance of the REM cycle (with respect to the sleep period) may be a causal factor in depression. The process that controls the REM cycle, however, is at present unknown. Further evidence that this phase advance is trait-like in depressives comes from studies of these patients while in remission (Hauri et al., 1974; Hauri & Hawkins, 1971), and a follow-up study of a nonpatient group that was reactively depressed during divorce (Cartwright, 1983). In all cases persons were studied while recovered and medication-free, yet the early REM latency was reported to persist, though at a more modest level. It is still speculative whether this sleep abnormality precedes the onset of an initial clinical episode. If so, this may be a useful marker of potential vulnerability. Sleep studies of persons at risk for depression, such as unaffected relatives of bioplar patients, should be done to clarify this issue.

Recently another aspect of the relation of circadian rhythm to depression has become a focus of research. It springs from the observation that some depressions are seasonal, as are suicides, and occur more often in the fall and winter when nights lengthen and daylight is reduced. The effect of light on entraining the human sleep-wake cycle is being studied intensively. One effect of light is to suppress melatonin; manic-depressive patients appear to be phase-advanced in their melatonin cycle in comparison to controls, and they also appear to be supersensitive to light. Lower levels of illumination will suppress melatonin in bipolars more than levels required to suppress normal controls. This has led to the use of light to reset the circadian rhythm as a therapeutic intervention for some depressed patients. Both Rosenthal et al. (1984) and Lewy (1983) report some success with this technique.

Although there has been good progress made in the past decade in understanding the nature of sleep disturbance in affective illness, there has been very little attention to the fact that it is specifically the sleep associated with dreaming that is affected. There are a few studies of dreams of the depressed and only one that tested specific hypotheses with respect to expected differences between the dreams of depressed and nondepressed persons (Trenholme et al., 1984).

DREAMS OF THE DEPRESSED

It would seem logical that if REM sleep is displaced from its normal position in the sleep cycle, occurring earlier and lasting longer on the first occasion, and being more active in terms of eye movement density, this might well be associated with disruptions in dreaming. Also, if distribution of REM sleep is changed from normal, across-the-night proportions and eye-movement density sequence is irregular, the whole nightly pattern of dream sequences may also differ from normal. Since dreaming appears to be intimately tied to affective experience and has been suggested to serve an adaptive problem-solving function, the phase-advance of REM sleep may be indicative of an abnormality in psychological processing of affective material.

There is some evidence to support the theory that dreams of depressed patients have less affect than dreams of normal controls. In fact, dreams of the depressed are reported to be bland and barren (Kramer et al., 1966) and do not become reinvested with affect until the depression begins to lift. At this time dream hostility and anxiety both increase (Kramer et al., 1968). These findings are also supported by a study that compared the dreams of two groups of women undergoing divorce; one group who became depressed, the other who did not. Only the dreams of the group who were not depressed showed anxiety increases across the night. Those who were depressed had increases in masochism in their dreams (Trenholme, et al., 1984). Masochism and dependency have both been associated with the dreams of the depressed in several studies (Beck & Ward, 1961; Kramer, et al., 1966; Hauri, 1976) and are two characteristics that appear to be more trait-like, reflecting stable aspects in dreams of reactive depressed patients even while they were in remission. Another aspect reported to be characteristic of dreams of the depressed is the tendency for dreams to be set in the past rather than in the present or future. Hauri (1976) reports this to be persistent in those remitted at least 6 months from a severe reactive episode that required hospitalization. Cartwright et al. (1984) also report dreams of depressed divorcees to be past-oriented in contrast to those of nondepressed or married controls. However, this aspect changed so that at a follow-up point 1–2 years later their dream time-frame was more variable and did not differ from controls.

Perhaps the most important of dream content findings from studies of the depressed that help to explain some of the treatment literature is the finding by Hauri (1976) that reactively depressed persons, when awakened from NREM sleep stages to give reports, "had excessive amounts of NREM thought." Their NREM reports were also often more dream-like than thought-like. This tendency for the reactively depressed to have overly active and dream-like mentation throughout their sleep stages may account for their failure to respond specifically to REM deprivation in the study by Vogel et al. (1975). Although the endogenous patients responded to the experimental condition of REM deprivation with improvement, they did not improve following the NREM awakening control condition. The reactive cases, however, responded equally well to both treatments. Vogel and colleagues interpreted this finding as a failure of the REM deprivation treatment for these patients and discontinued it for the reactive diagnostic group. It appears an equally tenable hypothesis that they responded to both awakening treatments (13 out of 18 improved) because both interrupted their dysfunctional cognitive patterns. Dwelling on the past, being masochistic and dependent, seeing the outside world as hostile, having negative motives, such as needs for abasement, and avoiding dealing with the present and future are all counterproductive for coping with realistic issues. REM-suppressing treatments carried out either by medication or by awakenings, whatever else their actions, also relieve the patient of this type of repetitive self-destructive thinking, at least temporarily. This may make patients more amenable to both psychotherapy and new ways of seeing themselves and the world when they awaken.

CONCLUSIONS

The depressed, whether bipolar or unipolar, inpatient or outpatient, endogenous or reactive, show REM sleep disturbances to various degrees. Primarily there is a phase advance of this rhythm, with respect to the sleep-wake rhythm, so that REM begins earlier, lasts longer, and is more active than in age-matched normals. Drugs of the tricyclic antidepressant or monoamine oxidase inhibitor (MOAI)-class both act to delay the first REM period and have the best chance of success in those patients who show this sign of shortened REM latency. An advantage of this drug effect on the sleep cycle is that it is predictive of clinical response almost immediately, although the change in mood and level of activation may take weeks to become manifest. That these drugs are efficacious to the extent that they reset the REM rhythm, with respect to the rest of sleep, is supported by the finding that remission can be accomplished without drugs by means of REM-depriving awakenings.

The nature of depressions is that they are repetitive, cyclic disorders. It appears that the tendency for the phase-advance of the REM system with respect to the sleep-wake rhythm does not remit completely between episodes. Since the dream content that accompanies REM also reveals some unremitting trait-like characteristics that can be characterized as inefficient patterns for dealing with the emotional impact of life events, it appears that depressive patients are vulnerable to future episodes unless there can be a reshaping of the affective–cognitive patterns as well. This could be encouraged by staff who are sensitive to these features of depressive illness: the tendency to self-blame, dwell on the past, and to be dependent and needy, while feeling unworthy. Care should be exercised by nursing personnel not to reinforce these attitudes when expressed but rather to ignore them and reinforce only present-oriented statements and independent actions. The staff also should be understanding of the sleep disruptions of these patients and willing to help them to deal with their distressing dream experiences in a calm and positive manner. Charting the sleep and noting when sleep loss is followed by clinical improvement would also be helpful to the treatment planning team.

REFERENCES

Aserinsky, E., & Kleitman, N. (1953). Regularly occurring periods of eye motility and concomitant phenomena during sleep. *Science, 118,* 237–274.

Beck, A., & Ward, C. (1961). Dreams of depressed patients: Characteristic themes in manifest content. *Archives of General Psychiatry, 5,* 462–467.

Cartwright, R. (1983). Rapid eye movement sleep characteristics during and after mood disturbing events. *Archives of General Psychiatry, 40,* 197–201.

Cartwright, R., Lloyd, S., Knight, S., & Trenholme, I. (1984). Broken dreams: A study of the effects of divorce and depression on dream content. *Psychiatry, 47,* 251–259.

Coble, P., Foster, G., & Kupfer, D. (1976). Electroencephalographic sleep diagnosis of primary depression. *Archives of General Psychiatry, 33,* 1124–1127.

Dement, W. (1960). The effect of dream deprivation. *Science, 131,* 1705–1707.

Dement, W., & Kleitman, N. (1957). The relation of eye movements during sleep to dream activity: An objective method for the study of dreaming. *Journal of Experimental Psychology, 53,* 339–346.

Duncan, W., Pettigrew, K., & Gillin, J. C. (1979). REM architecture changes in bipolar and unipolar depression. *American Journal of Psychiatry, 136,* 1424–1427,

Fahndrich, E. (1983). Effect of sleep deprivation as a predictor of treatment response to antidepressant medication. *Acta Psychiatrica Scandinavica, 68,* 341–344.

Feighner, J., Robins, E., & Guze, S. (1972). Diagnostic criteria for use in psychiatric research. *Archives of General Psychiatry, 26,* 57–63.

Feinberg, M., Gillin, J. C., Carroll, B., Greden, J., & Zis, A. (1982). EEG studies of sleep in the diagnosis of depression. *Biological Psychiatry, 17,* 305–316.

Gillin, J. C., Duncan, W., Pettigrew, K., Frankel, B., & Snyder, F. (1979). Successful separation of depressed, normal and insomniac subjects by EEG sleep data. *Archives of General Psychiatry, 36,* 85–90.

Hamilton, M. (1967). Development of a rating scale for primary depressive illness. *British Journal of Social Clinical Psychology.* 6: 278–296.

Hauri, P. (1976). Dreams in patients remitted from reactive depression. *Journal of Abnormal Psychology, 85,* 1–10.

Hauri, P., Chernik, D., Hawkins, D., & Mendels, J. (1974). Sleep of depressed patients in remission. *Archives of General Psychiatry, 31,* 386–391.

Hauri, P., & Hawkins, D. (1971). Phasic REM, depression and the relationship between sleeping and waking. *Archives of General Psychiatry, 25,* 56–63.

Kramer, M., Whitman, R., Baldridge, B., & Lansky, L. (1966). Dreaming in the depressed. *Canadian Psychiatric Association Journal, 11,* 178–192.

Kramer, M., Whitman, R., Baldridge, B., & Ornstein, P. (1968). Drugs and dreams. III. The effects of imipramine on the dreams of depressed patients. *American Journal of Psychiatry, 124,* 1385–1392.

Kripke, D., Mullaney, D., Atkinson, M., & Wolf, S. (1978). Circadian rhythm disorders in manic-depressives. *Biological Psychiatry, 13,* 335–351.

Kupfer, D., & Foster, G. (1972). Interval between onset of sleep and rapid eye movement sleep as an indicator of depression. *Lancet, 11,* 684–686.

Kupfer, D., & Foster, G. (1978). EEG sleep and depression. In R. Williams & I. Karacan (Eds.), *Sleep disorders: Diagnosis and treatment* (pp. 163-204). New York: John Wiley & Sons.

Kupfer, D., Foster, G., Reich, L., Thompson, K., & Weiss, B. (1976). EEG sleep changes as predictors in depression. *American Journal of Psychiatry, 133,* 622–626.

Lewy, A. (1983). Effects of light on melatonin secretion and the circadian system in man. In T. Wehr & F. Goodwin (Eds.), *Circadian rhythms in psychiatry* (pp. 203-220). Pacific Grove, Calif. Boxwood Press.

Rechtschaffen, A., & Kales, A. (1968). *A manual of standardized terminology, techniques and scoring for sleep stages of human subjects.* Washington, DC: U.S. Department of Health, Education and Welfare.

Reynolds, C., Newton, T., Shaw, D., Coble, P., & Kupfer, D. (1982). Electroencephalographic sleep findings in depressed outpatients. *Psychiatry Research, 6,* 65–75.

Rosenthal, N., Sack, D., Gillin, J. C., Lewy, A., Goodwin, F., Davenport, Y., Mueller, P., Newsome, D., & Wehr, T. (1984). Seasonal affective disorder. *Archives of General Psychiatry, 41,* 72–80.

Rush, A., Giles, D., Roffwarg, H., & Parker, R. (1982). Sleep EEG and dexamethasone suppression test findings in outpatients with unipolar major depressive disorders. *Biological Psychiatry, 17,* 327–341.

Svendsen, K., & Christensen, P. (1981). Duration of REM sleep latency as predictor of effect of antidepressant therapy. *Acta Psychiatrica Scandinavica, 64,* 238–243.

Taub, J., & Berger, R. (1975). The effects of changing the phase and duration of sleep. *Journal of Experimental Psychology, 2,* 30–41.

Trenholme, I., Cartwright, R., & Greenberg, G. (1984). Dream dimension differences during a life change. *Psychiatry Research.*

Vogel, G., Thurmond, A., Gibbons, P., Sloan, K., Boyd, M., & Walker, M. (1975). REM sleep reduction effects on depression syndromes. *Archives of General Psychiatry, 32,* 765–777.

Vogel, G., Vogel, F., McAbee, R., & Thurmond, A. (1980). Improvement of depression by REM sleep deprivation. *Archives of General Psychiatry, 37,* 247–253.

Webb, W., Agnew, H., & Williams, R. (1971). Effect on sleep of a sleep period time displacement. *Aerospace Medicine, 42,* 152–155.

Wehr, T., Gillin, J. C., & Goodwin, F. (in press). Sleep and circadian rhythms in depression. In M. Chase (Ed.), *New perspectives in sleep research.* New York: Spectrum Publishing.

Wehr, T., Muscettola, G., & Goodwin, F. (1980). Urinary MHPG circadian rhythm: Early timing (phase advance) in manic-depressives compared to normal subjects. *Archives of General Psychiatry, 37,* 257–263.

Wehr, T., Wirz-Justice, A., Goodwin, F., Duncan, W., & Gillin, J. C. (1979). Phase advance of the sleep–wake cycle as an antidepressant. *Science, 206,* 710–713.

Weitzman, E., Kripke, D., Goldmacher, D., McGregor, P., & Nogeire, C. (1970). Acute reversal of the sleep-wake cycle in man. *Archives of Neurology, 22,* 483–489.

Wirz-Justice, A., Puhringer, W., & Hole, G. (1976). Sleep deprivation and clomipramine in endogenous depression. *Lancet, 23,* 912.

	Electroconvulsive
	Therapy for the
6	Affectively Disordered
	Kathryn Gleason Cook

$\mathbf{T}$ he scenario is not a rarity: a severely depressed patient has not eaten for days, lies mute and virtually unresponsive to surroundings, becoming increasingly moribund. Electroconvulsive therapy (ECT) is started, often as a last resort, and within two or three days, the patient becomes responsive, starts eating, and begins recuperating. Despite such dramatic results, ECT remains a mysterious and dreaded therapeutic modality that is often misunderstood by consumers and professionals alike. But with increased knowledge of the physiological basis for ECT and the development of specific clinical protocols for its use, nurses now have the opportunity to create more rational approaches to the care of patients receiving ECT, especially to those with affective disorders.

PHYSIOLOGY OF ECT

Although incompletely defined, the physiological changes produced by ECT are now sufficiently well understood to allow the development of sophisticated hypotheses regarding ECT's specific action and to permit consideration of general explanatory schema unifying ECT with antidepressants and lithium as treatment modalities for affective disorders. Two concepts are central to this understanding: the immediate electrical effects of ECT and the likely role of hypothalamic activity in the psychopathology and treatment of affective disorders. Application of an adequate amount of electric current to the frontotemporal areas of the head produces immediate, but short-lived generalized electroencephalographic (EEG) changes within the brain—a seizure—and simultaneously, an observable tonic–clonic musculoskeletal reaction—a convulsion—easily identified as a grand mal convulsion. A generalized cerebral seizure is essential to the production of therapeutic results, whereas a convulsion is not (Freeman et al., 1978; Johnstone et al., 1980; Ottosson, 1960). Because ECT-induced convulsions may be hazardous to a patient's health and are frightening to experience or observe, in most protocols they have been chemically modified to the point of ablation without affecting the seizure.

ECT-induced electrical activity at the cerebral surface filters down through the brain structures until the hypothalamus, or at least the diencephalon is stimulated (Fink, 1979). Changes in plasma levels of several humoral substances subsequent to an ECT-induced seizure offer strong evidence for the hypothesis that ECT affects the hypothalamus itself. Immediate but transient increases can be demonstrated in ACTH, cortisol (Fink, 1982b), and prolactin levels (Arato et al., 1980; O'Dea et al., 1978), all of which are mediated by hypothalamic activity. With repeated electrical stimulation over time, more enduring effects of altered hypothalamic stimulation become evident. Clinical improvement (Maletzky, 1978), release of growth hormone (Gregoire et al., 1977; Kendler & Davis, 1977), and elevations in thyroid-stimulating hormone (Kirkegaard & Smith, 1978) and plasma prolactin (Coppen et al., 1980a), demonstrated after a series of ECT, strongly suggest substantial changes in hypothalamic-regulating functions. Such diverse effects of biochemical mediation by the hypothalamus are proposed to occur by the electrically induced release of several neuronal peptides affecting mood and behavior (Fink, 1979; Fink & Ottosson, 1980).

Another perspective provides data supporting the hypothalamic peptide hypothesis for ECT's specific therapeutic activity. Substantial evidence exists implicating hypothalamic dysfunction in psychopathologic states; if reverses in these dysfunctions can be demonstrated subsequent to ECT, support for the hypothesis obtains. Impaired hypothalamic activity is clearly manifested in the vegetative symptoms characteristic of the affective disorders: appetite disturbances, weight changes, sleep dysfunction, sexual behavior changes, and, in depression, decreased tear production, constipation, or amenorrhea (Fink, 1979; Fink & Ottosson, 1980; Haymaker et al., 1969). Additionally, specific neurochemical changes reflective of underlying hypothalamic dysfunction often accompany affective disorders, especially severe depression (Baldessarini, 1983). Two axes regulated by the hypothalamus have been of particular interest: hypothalamic-pituitary-adrenal (HPA) and hypothalamic-pituitary-thyroid (HPT).

A burgeoning literature describes a specific facet of HPA function in the affective disorders: that peripheral cortisol secretion is elevated in depression, fails to show its usual rhythmicity and, in some depressed persons is not suppressed by the oral administration of dexamethasone (Carroll et al., 1976a; 1976b), Thus, the dexamethasone suppression test (DST) acts as a peripheral biological marker for HPA activity (Carroll, 1982). It also showed promise for differentiating among subtypes of depression as well as predicting treatment outcome since ECT reversed the nonsuppression of cortisol by dexamethasone in anticipation of clinical improvement in some patients (Albala et al., 1981; Coryell, 1982). More recently, however, conflicting results have cast doubt on the ability of a simple procedure such as the DST to have such profound diagnostic and prognostic value (Coryell & Zimmerman, 1983; Decina et al., 1983; Haskett & Albala, 1982).

Similarly, studies of cortisol secretion in manic and hypomanic patients have yielded conflicting results with particular difficulties in distinguishing effects of arousal from those of manic illness or hormonal regulation (Ettigi & Brown, 1977). In manic-depressives, a lower level of cortisol secretion has been demonstrated in the manic phase than in the depressed phase (Stancer et al., 1969). These inconsistent and contradictory findings do not negate the significant, if complicated interplay of hypothalamic factors in the symptomatology and treatment of affective disorders. Rather, additional information is needed about ways in which the HPA axis is affected by pathology as well as ECT.

Less well-described, but nonetheless germane to an understanding of the affective disorders and their treatment, is the HPT axis. Normally, the hypothalamic peptide, thyrotropin-relasing hormone (TRH) increases plasma levels of thyroid-stimulating hormone (TSH) in a predictable temporal sequence (Grimm & Reichlin, 1973; Loosen & Prange, 1982). But in some severely depressed individuals, this effect is blunted (Gold et al., 1980; Kastin et al., 1972; Kirkegaard et al., 1975; Prange et al., 1972) and normalizes with recovery (Gregoire et al., 1977; Kirkegaard, & Smith, 1978; Linkowski et al., 1981) including those patients treated with ECT, suggesting as effect of treatment on the HPT axis itself. Some manics (Extein et al., 1980; Kirgegaard et al., 1978; Loosen & Prange, 1982) and alcoholics (Gold et al., 1981; Loosen & Prange, 1982) show similar findings. Thus the TSH response was viewed as a biological marker useful in making differential diagnoses (Asnis et al., 1980; Ehrensing et al., 1974; Gold et al., 1980) as well as predicting course and outcome of treatment (Kirkegaard, 1981) of the affectively disordered. Difficulties in replicating results after ECT (Coppen et al., 1980b; Deakin et al., 1983; Kirkegaard, 1981; Papakostas et al., 1981) along with methodological problems in test administration (Loosen & Prange, 1982) and definition of results (Haskett & Albala, 1982; Kirkegaard, 1981; Loosen & Prange, 1982) have thus far precluded the use of the TSH response in the clinical management of ECT patients. But because the modulation of TRH is clearly related to catecholamines implicated in affective disorders (Grimm & Reichlin, 1973), the potential importance of the HPT axis to an understanding of the pathophysiology and treatment of the affectively disordered cannot be ignored,

Thus far, it would then seem that the specific action of ECT involves the release of hypothalamic peptides, which in turn affect a variety of neural substrates, which ultimately affect behavior and mood states (Fink, 1979; Fink & Ottosson, 1980) as well as endocrine substances in the circulating plasma. From yet another perspective comes data suggesting that the major biochemical therapies for the affective disorders—tricyclic and monoamine oxidase inhibitors (MAIOs), antidepressants, lithium, and ECT—share common therapeutic mechanisms. Shifting from the effects of biological therapies on the production, release, uptake or reuptake of neurotransmitter substances to an examination of the effects of these same treatments on neurons has yielded interesting results.

Chronic administration of tricyclics and MAOIs results in decreased sensitivity of the beta-adrenergic receptors of post-synaptic neurons, occurring roughly at the same time clinical improvement is seen (Sachar, 1981). Repeated electrical convulsive shock (ECS) in animal models produces a similar reduction in beta-adrenergic receptor sensitivity (Lerer & Belmaker, 1982; Pand et al., 1979). While ECT and ECS are not precisely equivalent, the concordance is adequate for heuristic purposes. Lithium, on the other hand, is generally believed to stabilize receptor changes induced by other agents (Hermoni et al., 1980), perhaps accounting for its utility in preventing recurrent depressive or manic episodes. In similar fashion, ECT has been demonstrated to prevent changes in receptor sensitivity induced by haloperidol (Lerer & Belmaker, 1982). While this scanty evidence is far from convincing, it does present a clear possibility of the interrelated nature of the mechanisms of action of three treatment modalities heretofore believed quite different. Finally, one study found that antidepressants, lithium, and ECT all reduced the "total production of norepinephrine and/or its major metabolites" (Linnoila et al., 1983).

In summary then, specific action of ECT is believed to produce persistent release of substances, probably peptides, from the hypothalamus that mediates the peripheral endocrine, mood and behavioral changes observed when affectively disordered patients improve (Fink, 1979; Fink & Ottosson, 1980). Further, many of the specific neurochemical changes associated with successful ECT outcomes are similar to those identified with tricyclics, MAOIs, and even lithium (Linnoila et al., 1983).

SELECTION CRITERIA FOR ECT PATIENTS

Judicious use of ECT demands careful selection of potential candidates, somewhat analogous to the selection of medical patients for major surgical therapies. One effort designed to produce better matching of patients' symptomatologies with treatment modalities is the search for biological markers (i.e., neuroendocrine substances) in circulating blood. While many interesting and provocative linkages between clinical behaviors and biochemical processes have been identified, the imprecision of these relationships does not permit them to be the sole criterion for treatment decisions. As a result, the decision to use ECT remains an empirical one, albeit founded in substantial clinical diagnostic skill. The majority of patients believed to be appropriate for ECT are severely depressed, manifesting terminal insomnia, weight loss, psychomotor retardation or agitation, worsened symptomatology in the morning, and delusions of guilt, persecutory, or somatic content (American Psychiatric Association, 1978; Fink, 1979; Kendell, 1981; Scovern & Kilman, 1980; Taylor, 1982). Catatonic features respond especially well to ECT, regardless of diagnostic label (Fink, 1979; Taylor, 1982). ECT will also induce prompt improvement in actue manic episodes showing a wide range of symptomatology (Aden, 1976; McCabe, 1976; McCabe & Norris, 1977b; Taylor, 1982; Thomas & Reddy, 1982). Many patients just identified are treated biochemically in preference to ECT, either to avoid ECT-associated risks or because of other apprehensions about its use. Two exceptions are catatonics (Fink, 1979; Taylor, 1982) and depressives with somatic delusions or delusions of guilt; these patients clearly do not respond as well to medications as they do to ECT (Abrams & Taylor, 1977; Glassman et al., 1975; Kaskey et al., 1980; Rao & Coppen, 1979).

In the absence of clinically-independent biological predictors to differentiate between the remaining patients who need ECT and those who can be safely treated by other means, four clinical criteria can be used to appropriately select ECT candidates.

Lack of responsiveness to other treatment.   This defines a group of patients requiring ECT for relief of symptomatology. The most frequent contemporary use of ECT is to treat depressives who have not responded to one or more of the tricyclic antidepressants (Fink, 1982c; Kendell, 1981). Even patients who have not responded to a variety of antidepressants may obtain satisfactory symptom relief with ECT (Paul et al., 1981). It is probably less frequent that acutely ill manics fail to respond to some combination of lithium and neuroleptics, requiring ECT. Thus, no recent studies recommend ECT for treatment of actue mania because of failure to respond to other therapies. But it has been used successfully to treat manics who could not be maintained by lithium alone (Aden, 1976).

The time lag between initiation of treatment and the appearance of clinical improvement.   Time lag is a significant factor in the recommendation of ECT for some patients. Most antidepressants require 10–20 days to produce therapeutic results, whereas with ECT the same results can be seen in a few hours to 2–3 days (Coryell, 1978). Suicidal patients comprise the largest group clearly requiring prompt reversal of symptoms (American Psychiatric Association, 1978; Avery & Lubrano, 1979; Fink, 1979, 1982a; Scovern & Kilmann, 1980). Retrospective studies by Avery and Winokur (1976, 1978) indicate that even when antidepressants produce immediate reduction of suicidal behavior, the long-term suicidal rates are much greater for depressives treated with antidepressants than for those treated with ECT. Similarly, time-lag considerations also recommend the use of ECT for patients who are not taking adequate food or fluids because of their psychopathology (American Psychiatric Association, 1978; Kendell, 1981).

Differential tendencies of ECT and pharmacologic agents to precipitate physiological complications. These comprise a third set of factors supporting a decision to administer ECT. In general, the time span during which physiological side effects occur is much more limited for ECT than it is for antidepressants or antimania medications. With the exception of amnestic syndromes, most of the undesirable effects of ECT occur within minutes of the electrically-induced seizure (Bidder, 1981), permitting intensive supervision and external support of cardiorespiratory status until stability of vital signs has returned. Certainly, by one hour after ECT there is relatively little risk of developing life-threatening side effects. In contrast, undesirable effects of antidepressants, particularly in combination therapies, may occur at any time during the day, often have insidious beginnings with nearly fulminating consequences, and may persist for a considerable length of time. For patients who are likely to be at risk as a result of treatment side effects, ECT may be a much safer alternative.

ECT is also less likely to produce certain kinds of side effects than are antidepressants and antimanic drugs. For example, some cardiac arrhythmias, especially conduction defects, are almost certain to develop when tricyclics are utilized for susceptible cardiac patients (Jefferson, 1975); but ECT, if administered with appropriate anesthesia (Pitts, et al., 1965) and monitoring (Bidder, 1981; Pitts, 1982), does not produce these same effects. For other patients, particularly the elderly or medically ill, plasma tricyclic levels adequate to achieve clinical improvement cannot be attained without development of disabling orthostatic hypotension (Jefferson, 1975), or other arrhythmias (Bidder, 1981; Salzman, 1982), or both. Therefore, ECT is the most viable treatment alternative for these persons as well.

Tricyclics, lithium, and neuroleptics all have been found to cross the placental barrier with deleterious effects on the developing fetus (Ananth, 1975; Schou, 1980; Thomann & Hess, 1980; Thomas & Reddy, 1982). ECT, however, does not produce teratogenic effects, making it the treatment of choice for the pregnant depressed or manic individual, especially in the first trimester (Remick & Maurice, 1978). Further, the tendency of tricyclics to produce uncomfortable side effects has been suggested as a reason that nearly one-fifth of depressed outpatients treated with tricyclics discontinue their medication prematurely (Blackwell, 1982). ECT may also be a better treatment alternative for those depressed persons who cannot be relied on to continue the longer-term therapy needed with antidepressants.

Responsiveness to previous ECT. This makes a patient a prime candidate for ECT as the preferred treatment modality (Bidder, 1981; Taylor, 1982), regardless of whether or not the current episode has been treated with psychotropics. For such patients, disabling manifestations of untreated affective disorders together with the likely complications of pharmacologic therapies tilt the risk-benefit ratio in favor of ECT. A family history of a positive response to ECT for a similar set of symptoms in a blood relative is also a good indicator that ECT should be treatment of choice (Bidder, 1981). ECT remains then a therapeutic modality useful in treating patients who have severe affective illness that is unresponsive to psychotropics, who cannot be safely managed during the time-lag needed for medications to be effective, who cannot tolerate or risk side effects of pharmacologic therapies, or who have previously achieved a remission of symptoms with ECT.

INDICATORS OF POSITIVE RESPONSE TO ECT

Positive response to ECT can be clearly identified by nursing staff who are familiar with effects of hypothalamic stimulation as well as a patient's unique behavioral manifestations of affective disorder. Early signs of a positive response to ECT are to be found in the vegetative behaviors accompanying depression or mania. In either case, the earliest sign of improvement subsequent to ECT is likely to be found in nighttime sleep behaviors. Most commonly, the length of time a patient sleeps before awakening with intermittent or terminal insomnia will increase noticeably (i.e., one hour or more), but not to the point of having uninterrupted sleep. A simple way of documenting these changes is to keep sleep records, recording sleep status at least every 30 minutes. Such changes may occur after the first ECT, but are more likely to be seen after the second and third treatments. Even so, nighttime sleep on nonECT days may not improve until the fifth or sixth treatment.

For depressed patients, other early signs of improvement involve eating behaviors. Particularly for the first meal eaten after receiving ECT, patients are likely to show an increase in the amount of food eaten, whether they are able to eat independently or not. Beginning to eat may still be difficult to establish, but once eating is started, more food is ingested. Early in the treatment series, this effect may be particularly transient, so that a return to previous eating behaviors will occur within a few hours. As the ECT series progresses to the third or fourth treatment, this effect begins to stabliize and generalize to other meals of the day.

Carbohydrate craving is often associated with ECT-induced improvement, reflecting hypothalamic stimulation. This interesting behavior takes many forms, some of which staff find problematic in milieu management. Surreptitious gulping of candy, cookies, ice cream and, other sweets is not uncommon, even in patients who still have major deficits in concentration and verbalization. Typically, carbohydrate craving is at its peak from the second or third treatment through the fifth or sixth, and gradually subsides after the treatment series ends. Often, patients do not recall and even flatly deny this aspect of their recovery in subsequent conversations. Decisions about the management of these behaviors need to be based on an understanding of the nutritional, milieu, and other medical issues affecting a patient.

The last of the eating behaviors to manifest improvement is appetite; that is, patients' reports of feeling hungry, or having a desire to eat, or both. Lack of appetite may persist despite well-established increases in amounts of food ingested and rarely disappears in depressed patients prior to the fourth or fifth treatment. Initially, return of appetite will be a transient effect also, showing regression within 24 hours or less, but generally stabilizes as the treatment series is completed. Once eating is re-established however, most patients will increase their food intake despite the lack of appetite they experience.

It is not as easy to generalize about the early indicators of improvement in manic patients. Eating behaviors do not seem to be as specifically affected, nor do they change as quickly as they do for depressed persons. Rather, more subtle improvements in a variety of behaviors involving impulse control are likely to be seen, usually manifested in a gradual need for fewer p.r.n. medications, time-outs, or whatever other methods are used to contain impulsive behavior. Sometimes, manic patients begin to do more daytime sleeping, especially in response to neuroleptic medications. Frank, sexual acting-out is likely to decrease long before verbalizations of sexual content disappear from a manic's repertoire.

Arousal of anger is a later indicator of clinical improvement seen in some depressed patients, usually about the fourth or fifth treatment, and lasting until the series ends, or shortly thereafter. A variety of angry behaviors may be exhibited, including swearing, yelling, and making disparaging remarks about specific significant others. In many cases, these angry behaviors appear to have a cathartic effect, resulting in a more calm patient after their expression. Beneficial effects of the arousal are not diminished by channeling the associated energy into less direct forms of physical expression such as exercise, craft projects, and active games. Patients who experience this angry arousal usually do not recall either the experience or their related behaviors when interviewed several days or weeks after completing the ECT series.

Verbalization of a subjective sense of improvement is the last indicator of a positive response to ECT to appear in recovery of either manics or depressives. Direct questioning may not yield a positive response until the series is completed, or even later in some patients. Occasionally, the difficulty in obtaining a positive statement of subjective improvement is associated with frank denial of the illness episode. This may be particularly true in instances where short-term memory loss accompanies ECT. In other circumstances, lack of sense of subjective improvement is thought to reflect a mixed presentation of psychopathology, only part of which was amenable to ECT, and requiring subsequent pharmacologic treatment as well. Whatever the situation, clinicians need to be able to gauge improvement using a set of observable criteria rather than relying entirely on self-reports of improvement.

ADVERSE EFFECTS OF ECT

Adverse effects actually or purportedly attribued to ECT are frequently identified by clinicians and lay person alike as factors important in the resistance to its use. Chief among these effects is ECT-related memory loss, described in a large and very complex literature of clinical and experimental studies from which few practical guides for clinical practice can be derived. Memory is a difficult cognitive function to assess (American Psychiatric Association, 1978; Price, 1982a; Squire, 1982) often requiring technological measurements yielding data that are not easily translated into clinical practice issues (for example, paired-associates learning tasks are not closely analogous to social learning situations in which inpatients find themselves). Also, objective measures of memory function may not corroborate one's subjective experience of memory loss, and despite knowledge that ECT and depression differentially affect immediate retention and forgetting (Cronholm & Ottosson, 1961; Stromgren, 1977), only recently have systematic attempts been made to distinguish ECT-induced memory loss from that related to pre-existing illnesses (Squire et al., 1979; Sternberg & Jarvik, 1976; Wexler, 1980).

Two features of ECT-induced memory loss are most significant to clinicians: types of memory deficit and the temporal sequence over which they occur. Both anterograde and retrograde amnesia can be induced by ECT, using contemporary protocols. Anterograde amnesia, the inability to transfer newly learned material into long-term memory (Price, 1982a), may be produced by either bilateral or unilateral ECT (d'Elia, 1970; Fleminger et al., 1970; Halliday et al., 1968), but bilateral results in more anterograde amnesia than does unilateral nondominant (American Psychiatric Association, 1978; Lancaster et al., 1958) or unilateral dominant ECT (Jackson, 1978) when verbal memory function is measured (Daniel & Crovitz, 1983b; Price, 1982a). When the effects of bilateral and unilateral ECT on nonverbal memory aspects of anterograde amnesia have been measured, mixed findings resulted (Daniel & Crovitz, 1983b; Price, 1982a). Neither are the effects of electrical stimulus modality (sinusoidal or brief-pulse) on amount of anterograde amnesia clear-cut (Daniel & Crovitz, 1983a; Price, 1982a). Anterograde amnesia does appear to be worse for events learned temporally closer to ECT than those learned farther away (Price, 1982b; Squire et al., 1976). Recovery from anterograde amnesia is believed to be "considerably" recovered 1 month post-ECT (Squire, 1982) and nearly complete

6–9 months after the series ends (American Psychiatric Association, 1978; Price, 1982a; Squire, 1982).

Retrograde amnesia, an inability to recall events occurring prior to ECT (Price, 1982a), is a memory deficit most familiar to clinicians working with ECT patients. An interesting example is found with bilingual patients, particularly those who have learned English as a second language in adulthood, and who after a series of ECT, will temporarily forget their second language, reverting to their native tongues until the amnesia recedes. Both bilateral and unilateral ECT produce retrograde amnesia (Cohen et al., 1968), but bilateral produces significantly more than either form of unilateral ECT (Daniel & Crovitz, 1983b; d'Elia, 1970; Price, 1982a; Squire, 1982). A temporal gradient exists for ECT-induced retrograde amnesia so that events occurring nearest ECT are forgotten earliest and recall of those events, whether public or autobiographical in nature, will be last to return (American Psychiatric Association, 1978; Price, 1982a; Squire, 1975; Squire et al., 1980). Recall of the temporal order of events is particularly sensitive to ECT-induced amnesia (Squire et al., 1976) and may be impaired for sequential information learned several years prior to treatment (Squire, 1977). Amount of retrograde amnesia is positively related to the number and frequency of treatments (Dornbush et al., 1971; Fromholt et al., 1973; Squire & Miller, 1974), but is not likely to be related to stimulus type (i.e., sinusoidal or brief-pulse) used for ECT (Daniel & Crovitz, 1983a; Spanis & Squire, 1981; Weaver et al., 1977). The memory deficit in retrograde amnesia tends to be spotty rather than all-or-none (Squire, 1982), and recedes spontaneously after an ECT series is completed (American Psychiatric Association, 1978; Price, 1982a; Squire, 1982). Although recovery is believed to be reasonably complete by 6–9 months post-ECT (American Psychiatric Association, 1978; Price, 1982a; Squire, 1982), memory for some events surrounding the ECT series may be permanently lost (American Psychiatric Association, 1978; Price, 1982a; Squire, 1982),resulting in what patients sometimes call annoying ''gaps'' in memory that do not impair their overall function (Freeman et al., 1980; Taylor et al., 1982).

The temporal sequence in which ECT-induced memory deficits develop can be divided into four phases: post-ictal (immediately following each treatment), inter-ictal (between treatments, but not inclusive of the immediate post-ictal period), post-treatment (after the ECT series has been completed, but not inclusive of the last post-ictal period), and long-term (usually arbitrarily defined as 6 months post-ECT and beyond). Obviously, the demarcation of these periods has much more conceptual than clinical clarity. Nonetheless, some significant differences in clinical manifestations can be described. Memory impairment in the post-ictal period is apparent immediately upon recovery and persists for a variable amount of time, depending on type of anesthesia used (Fink, 1979), number and frequency of treatments (Dornbush et al., 1971; Fromholt et al., 1973; Miller, 1970; Zubin, 1948), and whether unilateral or bilateral ECT is used (d'Elia, 1970; Fink, 1979, Squire, 1982). Occasionally, the onset of post-ictal memory impairment may be delayed up to 24 hours (Hargreaves et al., 1972). Post-ictal memory deficits tend to be retrograde, fairly limited in scope and last from approximately 45 minutes early in the series (Squire et al., 1978) to several hours after the sixth or eighth treatments (Goldman et al., 1972; Squire et al., 1975).

Inter-ictal memory deficits include both retrograde and anterograde amnesia. Anterograde amnesia recedes rapidly after each treatment early in the series, but tends to accumulate as the series progresses (Daniel & Crovitz, 1983a; Price, 1982a; Squire & Miller, 1974) so that early in the series, patients may demonstrate relatively few anterograde deficits late in the inter-ictal period if they did not have anterograde deficits prior to starting ECT. Retrograde amnesia develops more gradually but persistently than anterograde; thus, by the fifth or sixth treatment, retrograde amnesia is well-established throughout most of the inter-ictal period (Squire, 1975). By the end of a typical bilateral ECT series (six or eight treatments), patients will show both significant anterograde and retrograde deficits.

Clearing of the last post-ictal period marks the beginning of the post-treatment phase, which is characterized by pronounced anterograde and retrograde amnesia in the beginning. Spontaneous recovery of anterograde amnesia is usually evident one week posttreatment and is "considerably" complete by one month (Squire, 1982). Retrograde amnesia clears more slowly, along the temporal gradient previously described, but even with bilateral ECT is showing improvement by the end of the second post-ECT week (American Psychiatric Association, 1978). During the post-treatment period, patients show gradual improvement in memory function until an asymptote is reached, signalling the beginning of the long-term phase.

Long-term memory deficits induced by ECT have attracted much interest and study, but are difficult to describe because of a myriad of methodological problems (Taylor et al., 1982), including much difficulty in attributing causality to the deficits that persist post-ECT. Spotty retrograde amnesia is characteristically present with patients' subjective reports of memory impairment exceeding objectively demonstrable defects (Freeman et al., 1980; Johnstone et al., 1980; Squire & Chace, 1975; Squire et al., 1980; Weeks et al., 1980). This interesting relationship is associated with some other types of amnesia as well (Kahn et al., 1975) and is not characteristic of all ECT patients (Kendell, 1981; Squire, 1982). Most conclude that the enduring memory deficits of this period are irritating but not incapacitating (Kendell, 1981; Squire, 1982; Taylor et al., 1982). Nursing assessments of long-term memory deficits, as well as those of earlier phases, need to be based on knowledge of an individual's pre-treatment function along with anticipated behaviors throughout the treatment sequence. In particular, careful assessment is required to move beyond stereotypic responses that may mask either anterograde or retrograde deficits.

Other cognitive deficits often associated with ECT are confusion and disorientation. Frequently ECT-related research has not adequately differentiated between these two states, making comparative statements difficult. Both are characteristic of the post-ictal period and to a lesser extent, the inter-ictal period. Confusion is generally described as the more global function, sometimes dependent on disorientation for definition (Daniel & Crovitz, 1982). Global estimates of confusion are usually evident for 30–40 minutes after each bilateral treatment (Squire, 1982), but are considerably diminished in intensity or duration after unilateral nondominant ECT (Fraser & Glass, 1980; Impastato & Karlinger, 1966; Lancaster et al., 1958). Likewise, sinusoidal stimulation is more likely to produce confusion than is brief-pulse ECT (Cronholm & Ottosson, 1963; Valentine et al., 1968).

ECT-induced disorientation and its recovery have been much more precisely described insofar as sequence is concerned, but the exact time of recovery of orientation remains variable depending on such variables as type of anesthesia and oxygenation method used for ECT (Daniel & Crovitz, 1982). Recovery of orientation always proceeds from person to place to time (d'Elia, 1970; Gottlieb & Wilson, 1965; Mowbray, 1954) and occurs more rapidly in unilateral than bilateral ECT (d'Elia, 1970; Fraser & Glass, 1978; Halliday et al., 1968; Lancaster et al., 1958; Wilson & Gottlieb, 1967). Unlike unilateral ECT, the amount of time to recover orientation has been found to increase for bilateral as the ECT series progresses (Fraser & Glass, 1978). Finally, sinusoidal stimulation is believed to prolong the time to regain orientation more than does brief-pulse ECT (Daniel & Cravitz, 1982). Clearly, the cognitive deficits associated with ECT have significant implications for nurses' expectations regarding patients' behaviors, appropriate patient education, and management of milieu issues that may arise.

In a limited number of cases, an acute organic brain syndrome or delirium may develop post-ECT and clear suddenly after a number of hours or days (Fink, 1979; Kalinowsky, 1945; Marshall et al., 1980). More recently, a large percentage of these cases has been attributed to an interaction between anticholinergic medications and ECT (Mondimore et al., 1983; Summers et al., 1979). For some, but not all patients, the interaction of lithium and ECT and/or its chemical modifiers produces a similar delirious state (Hoenig & Chaulk, 1977; Mandel et al., 1980; Small et al., 1980; Weiner et al., 1980). In either case, the dynamics of the proposed interactions are only sketchily described.

Much more frequently, patients will experience headache subsequent to ECT in the post-ictal and early inter-ictal phases. One-third to one-half of ECT patients are believed to have post-seizure headaches (Abrams, 1982; Freeman & Kendell, 1980; Hughes et al., 1981) that are relieved by mild analgesics such as acetaminophen or aspirin. There is conflicting evidence as to whether bilateral or unilateral ECT produces headache more frequently or of greater intensity (Fraser & Glass, 1980; Gomez, 1975). Certainly, if ECT patients are affected with significant memory deficits, assessment of headache should be based on nonverbal behaviors suggesting such an underlying state, as well as verbal responses to specific questioning.

When ECT is used to treat patients with a bipolar affective disorder, there is always a risk that treatment will precipitate either a hypomanic episode for depressed patients or a depressive episode for manic patients. This is particularly likely to occur if ECT is combined with concurrent antidepressant therapy (Siris et al., 1982). In either case, careful clinical assessment is required after each individual treatment, recognizing that normally the initial effects of the treatment on mood and behavior tend to decay over time as the inter-ictal phase progresses. This decay does not occur when these iatrogenic hypomanic or depressive episodes are precipitated, and behaviors observed tend to be reminiscent of prior episodes patients have experienced. Discontinuing ECT may be sufficient to interrupt the new episode, or for some patients additional therapy, including carbamazepine may be required to stabilize mood and behavior.

In summary, adverse effects of ECT primarily involve temporary deficits in memory and/or orientation and post-seizure headache. Less frequently, significant temporary confusional states develop. In a few vulnerable patients, delirium and depressive or hypomanic episodes can be produced subsequent to ECT.

NURSING IMPLICATIONS OF SPECIFIC ECT PROTOCOLS

Four types of protocols have specific implications for nursing practice with ECT patients: chemical modification of ECT, electrode placement, modifications for the medically ill, and special protocols for the elderly. This discussion will be limited to those issues occurring either pre-ECT, or after recovery from anesthesia. Several protocols for chemical modification have been described in detail (Abrams, 1982; Fink, 1979; Pitts, 1982) and routinely include use of anticholinergic agents to achieve vagal blockade, general anesthesia, and skeletal muscle blockade. Anticholinergic agents may be given subcutaneously or intramuscularly 30–45 minutes pre-ECT with results and implications analogous to other preoperative patients. However, it may be preferable to administer the anticholinergic agent intravenously just prior to application of ECT electrodes, particularly if peripheral circulation is compromised in some way. Because atropine crosses the blood–brain barrier, it may be more likely to be associated with post-ECT delirium, causing alternative compounds to be selected (Pitts, 1982).

The most frequently selected anesthetic agents are thiopental sodium and methohexital, with methohexital being preferred as it is less likely to be associated with cardiac arrhythmias (Pitts et al., 1965). However, if thiopental sodium is used for ECT, patients are more likely to remain sleepy after recovery from anesthesia, requiring specific supervision of activity and other safety measures. Succinylocholine is the most frequently used skeletal muscle relaxant (Fink,

1979; Pitts, 1982), but precise dosage for each patient may require some titration across the series of treatments. If slightly less than ideal amounts of succinylcholine have been used for a single treatment, staff can expect that a patient might experience mild muscle aching during the early inter-ictal period. This aching is usually noticed in neck and shoulder musculature and can be relieved with mild analgesia, or warm moist packs, or both.

Electrode placement for the actual application of ECT has far-reaching implications for nursing care of patients post-ECT. As described earlier, bilateral stimulation, usually delivered bitemporally, will produce anterograde and retrograde amnesia, and is more likely to be associated with disorientation and confusion. All of these effects require not only careful assessment but also vigilant intervention by nursing staff to ensure safety and maintain optimal functioning of post-ECT patients. Establishment of realistic and predictable expectations of patients, reliable routines of daily activity, and ongoing assessment of physiologic status are essential for patients during times when they may have difficulty organizing and communicating their experiences as well as remembering information communicated to them. Some studies (Price, 1982a) suggest that prompting or use of specific focusing techniques may assist the spontaneous clearing of retrograde amnesia. Reorientation and remotivation activities already familiar to psychiatric nurses' practices may be useful in this regard.

Sequelae of unilateral ECT vary considerably with the exact placement of unilateral electrodes. In general, patients have less difficulty with amnesia, disorientation, and confusion than do those receiving bilateral ECT. Headaches post-ECT tend to be localized to the stimulated hemisphere, which is an unfamiliar and worrisome experience for some patients. Occasionally, patients treated with unilateral ECT may experience an incomplete seizure (Fink et al., 1958), resulting in a failure to stimulate diencephalic areas. Clinically, this tends to be manifested by an initial subjective sense of having been "stunned" along with a dull headache that is responsive to analgesics. More importantly, as the inter-ictal period progresses, a lack of clinical improvement becomes evident. Precise monitoring of seizure activity during the treatment itself helps decrease the likelihood of these incomplete seizures (Welch, 1982). There is also some evidence that clinical improvement will require more treatments using the unilateral mode (Abrams et al., 1972; Reichert et al., 1976), in the range of two or three treatments more than would be expected for a bilateral series.

Although the efficacy of unilateral and bilateral ECT is roughly equivalent (American Psychiatric Association, 1978), there is, however, a subset of patients,—as yet poorly defined,—who do not respond to unilateral treatment, and thus require bilateral ECT (Abrams et al., 1973; 1983; Price, 1981). These patients are usually identified by their lack of clinical improvement only as the unilateral series progresses. Changing to bilateral treatment can be accomplished without any changes in pre-treatment protocols. Finally, there are some patients for whom the risk of not responding to unilateral ECT is simply too great to consider anything other than bilateral stimulation. Suicidal and catatonic patients (Abrams, 1982) are prominent in this group.

Because there are no medical conditions that absolutely contradict the use of ECT (Abrams, 1982; Fink, 1979; Small & Small, 1981), and at the same time, many more medically ill patients are candidates for ECT (Bidder, 1981), nurses can anticipate the need to modify either preparation or aftercare for ECT for a significant number of patients. Detailed assessment of a variety of baseline data is critical to the safe administration of ECT in the medically ill, including cardiovascular and respiratory function in all medically ill patients and insulin regulation in diabetes. For the medically ill, anticholinergic medication is more likely to be given intravenously (Bidder, 1981), but otherwise no specific pre-treatment is recommended for most patients who are likely to experience cardiovascular complications during the treatment itself (Elliott et al., 1982; Gerring & Shields, 1982; Pitts, 1982). An exception is pacemaker patients for whom it is desirable to x-ray for precise electrode placement prior to beginning an ECT series (Abiuso, et al., 1978; Alexopoulos & Frances, 1980); it may also be desirable to omit anticholinergic medication as well (Alexopoulos & Frances, 1980). Patients on anticoagulant therapy may be maintained on warfarin sodium or changed to minidose heparin therapy during an ECT series (Alexopoulos et al., 1982; Elliott et al., 1982). Diabetics often experience altered insulin requirements during a course of ECT (Elliott et al., 1982; Small & Small, 1981), either as a direct result of ECT on the HPA axis, or indirectly from changes in behavior subsequent to ECT, or both. In either case, diabetics often require more frequent assessment of endocrine status and titration of insulin dosage. Finally, for some medically ill patients, bilateral ECT may be recommended to reduce the number of exposures to ECT and its chemical modifiers (Bidder, 1981). If such a course is selected, all of the aforementioned cognitive deficits can be anticipated post-ECT in addition to behavioral correlates of a patient's usual medical condition.

Elderly depressed patients are more likely to both require and respond to ECT and yet have special needs following treatment. Recovery from each individual treatment takes longer in the elderly (Fraser & Glass, 1978; 1980) and is more likely to be associated with cognitive deficits that subjectively (Gomez, 1975) and objectively (Pettinati & Bonner, 1984) take longer to clear. Further, bilateral ECT is much more likely than unilateral to produce these adverse effects (Fraser & Glass, 1978; Salzman, 1982). Thus, a recommended protocol for the elderly is to administer unilateral treatments twice weekly (Salzman, 1982; Small & Small, 1981) to permit maximal clearing of cognitive deficits in the inter-ictal period. Unfortunately, some elderly patients do not respond well to unilateral ECT, requiring the use of bilateral (Salzman, 1982) and its concomitant implications for nursing care. In addition, older people experience a great deal more unsteadiness of gait or frank ataxia (Fraser & Glass, 1980) than do younger persons post-ECT. Whether this is a result of ECT and its cognitive effects, anesthesia, or some combination of factors is unclear. What is quite evident from clinical practice, however, is that elderly patients are exquisitely prone to falling in the early inter-ictal period post-ECT.

PREPARATION OF PATIENTS AND FAMILIES FOR ECT

Physical preparation of patients for ECT is not unlike that for minor surgical procedures, and in some institutions it may be identical. Protocols specific for ECT (Abrams, 1982; Fink, 1979) usually include chest and spine films with basic blood work and urinalysis. Patients are maintained on NPO status the night prior to each treatment, which may require some creative nursing management on typical inpatient psychiatric units. Voiding prior to ECT prevents discomfort immediately post-ECT, but failure to void will usually not result in incontinence during the treatment. As with surgical procedures, signed consent is necessary for the treatment series. In addition, a variety of legal issues surround the use of ECT in contemporary America (American Psychiatric Association, 1978; Frankel, 1982), requiring careful consideration prior to beginning a treatment sequence.

Emotional preparation for ECT is also similar to that needed prior to any procedure requiring general anesthesia. In addition, some patients may experience fears specifically related to ECT itself along with frightening symptomatology associated with the presenting illness. Supportive interventions and/or p.r.n. anxiolytic agents usually will assist patients in dealing with their psychic distress. It is helpful for nurses to address four areas in an assessment of a patient's reaction to a decision to use ECT and resultant preparations: (1) what the meaning of the illness is to the patient; (2) what effect the patient expects ECT to have on the illness; (3) what the patient's expectation is about the experience of ECT itself; (4) and, what effect the present illness has on the patient's ability to process and remember information. Finally, nurses need to be keenly aware of their own beliefs and affective responses to ECT in general, as well as its specific prescription for the patient in question, in order to better understand the effects of those beliefs and reactions on the nursing care provided.

Families typically have several needs prior to and during a course of ECT. Education regarding ECT's therapeutic rationale, preparation, and aftercare frequently is needed or desired by significant others in addition to information provided by physicians. During the course of ECT, family members often need support while experiencing a patient's cognitive deficits and/or behavioral reactions. It is not unusual that these are not only worrisome to family members, but are perceived to be so ego-alien as to be overwhelming. If a patient has temporary cognitive deficits, there may be a need to assist significant others in discerning clinical improvement that may be obscured by amnesia, disorientation, or confusion. Lastly, if either psychopathology or ECT-related cognitive deficits have interrupted usual communication patterns between significant others and an ECT patient, both education and direct intervention to promote communication may be needed from staff.

MAINTENANCE AND OUTPATIENT ECT

More controversial uses of ECT are to maintain the therapeutic gains achieved from an ECT series and/or to treat depressed outpatients. Maintenance ECT consists of the administration of single treatments spaced at increasing time intervals (for example, one week, then two weeks, then five weeks, then two months) after a traditional series is completed, usually on an outpatient basis. Conflicting evidence exists as to whether or not maintenance ECT actually reduces relapses (Barton et al., 1973; Karliner & Wehrheim, 1965); that may be due, in part, to a difficulty in differentiating relapses from new episodes of affective illness (Haskett, 1982). Nonetheless, it may be a reasonable contemporary alternative for patients who cannot be maintained with antidepressants or lithium (Abrams, 1982; Kendell, 1981) or for the elderly (Fink, 1979) or medically ill who cannot tolerate effects of drug therapy. Maintenance therapy is not recommended on an indefinite basis because of the possibility of cognitive deficits developing with increasing numbers of ECT (Abrams, 1982).

Outpatient ECT is comparable in many respects to minor one-day surgical procedures. Patients usually stay in the treatment unit for 2–3 hours after initial recovery from anesthesia, then are released to the care of a significant other. The ability to resume usual daily activies is an individual matter, determined in part by the very nature of those activities. A potential problem area with maintenance ECT is assuring that NPO status has been maintained prior to each treatment, and may require a variety of nursing interventions with the patient and significant others. In a few instances, outpatient unilateral ECT has been used exclusively to treat depressives in a traditional series (Abrams, 1982).

SUMMARY

ECT is an appropriate biological therapy useful with specific kinds of affective disorders and in some instances may be the treatment of choice. Nursing assessment is a significant aspect of the data base from which a decision to use ECT, as well as determination of therapeutic response or adverse effects, is made. Specific implications for nursing care can be derived from patient and family characteristics, specific protocols, and knowledge of the physiological basis for ECT.

REFERENCES

Abiuso, P., Dunkelman, R., & Proper, M. (1978). Electroconvulsive therapy in patients with pacemakers. *Journal of the American Medical Association, 224*, 2459–2460.

Abrams, R. (1982). Technique of electroconvulsive therapy. In R. Abrams & W. B. Essman (Eds.), *Electroconvulsive therapy*. New York: Spectrum Publications, pp. 41–55.

Abrams, R., Fink, M., Dornbush, R. L., Feldstein, S., Volavka, J., & Roubicek, J. (1972). Unilateral and bilateral ECT: Effects on depression, memory and the electroencephalogram. *Archives of General Psychiatry, 27*, 88–91.

Abrams, R., Fink, M., & Feldstein, S. (1973). Prediction of clinical response to ECT. *British Journal of Psychiatry, 122*, 457–460.

Abrams, R., & Taylor, M. A. (1977). Catatonia: Prediction of response to somatic treatments. –American Journal of Psychiatry, 134, 70–80.

Abrams, R., Taylor, M. A., Faber, R., Ts'o, T. O. T., Williams, R. A., & Almy, G. (1983). Bilateral versus unilateral electroconvulsive therapy in melancholia. *American Journal of Psychiatry, 140*, 463–465.

Aden, G. C. (1976). Lithium carbonate vs. ECT in the treatment of the manic state of identical twins with bipolar affective disease. *Diseases of the Nervous System, 37*, 393–397.

Albala, A. A., Greden, J. F., Tarika, J., & Carroll, B. J. (1981). Changes in serial dexamethasone suppression tests among unipolar depressives receiving electroconvulsive treatment. *Biological Psychiatry, 16*, 551–560.

Alexopoulos, G. S., & Frances, R. J. (1980). ECT and cardiac patients with pacemakers. *American Journal of Psychiatry, 137*, 1111–1112.

Alexopoulos, G. S., Nasr, H., Young, R. C., Wikstrom, T. R., & Holzman, S. R. (1982). Electroconvulsive therapy in patients on anticoagulants. *Canadian Journal of Psychiatry, 27*, 46–48.

American Psychiatric Association. (1978). Electroconvulsive therapy (Task Force Report #14). Washington, D.C.: American Psychiatric Association.

Ananth, J. V. (1975). Congenital malformations with psychopharmacologic agents. *Comprehensive Psychiatry, 16*, 436–445.

Arato, M., Erdos, A., Kurcz, M., Vermes, I., & Fekete, M. (1980). Studies on the prolactin response induced by electroconvulsive therapy in schizophrenics. *Acta Psychiatrica Scandinavia, 61*, 239–244.

Asnis, G. M., Nathan, R. S., Halbreich, U., Halpern, F. S. & Sachar, E. J. (1980). TRH tests in depression. *Lancet, 1*, 424–425.

Avery, D., & Lubrano, A. (1979). Depression treated with imipramine and ECT: The de Carolis study reconsidered. *American Journal of Psychiatry, 136*, 559–562.

Avery, D., & Winokur, G. (1976). Mortality in depressed patients treated with electroconvulsive therapy and antidepressants. *Archives of General Psychiatry, 33*, 1029–1037.

Avery, D., & Winokur, G. (1978). Suicide, attempted suicide, and relapse rate in depression. *Archives of General Psychiatry, 35*, 749–753.

Baldessarini, R. J. (1983). *Biomedical aspects of depression and its treatment*. Washington, D.C.: American Psychiatric Press.

Barton, J. L., Mehta, S., & Snaith, R. P. (1973). The prophylactic value of extra ECT in depressive illness. *Acta Psychiatric Scandinavica, 49,* 386–392.

Bidder, T. G. (1981). Electroconvulsive therapy in the medically ill patient. *Psychiatric Clinics of North America, 4,* 391–405.

Blackwell, B. (1982). Antidepressant drugs: Side effects and compliance. *Journal of Clinical Psychiatry, 43,* (1, Sec. 2), 14–18.

Carroll, B. J. (1982). Use of the dexamethasone suppression test in depression. *Journal of Clinical Psychiatry, 43,* (11, Sec. 2), 44–48.

Carroll, B. J., Curtis, H. G., & Mendels, J. (1976a). Neuroendocrine regulation in depression. I. Limbic system-adrenocortical dysfunction. *Archives of General Psychiatry, 33,* 1039–1044.

Carroll, B. J., Curtis, H. G., & Mendels, J. (1976b). Neuroendocrine regulation in depression. II. Discrimination of depressed persons from nondepressed patients. *Archives of General Psychiatry, 33,* 1051–1058.

Cohen, B. D., Noblin, C. D., Silverman, A. J., & Penick, S. B. (1968). Functional asymmetry of the human brain. *Science, 162,* 475–476.

Coppen, A., Rao, V. A. R., Bishop, M., Abou-Saleh, M., & Wood, K. (1980a). Neuroendocrine studies in affective disorders. Part 1. Plasma prolactin response to thyrotropin-releasing hormone in affective disorders: Effect of ECT. *Journal of Affective Disorders, 2,* 311–315.

Coppen, A., Rao, V. A. R., Bishop, M., Abou-Saleh, M., & Wood, K. (1980b). Neuroendocrine studies in affective disorders. Part 2. Plasma thyroid-stimulating hormone response to thyrotropin-releasing hormone in affective disorders: Effect of ECT. *Journal of Affective Disorders, 2,* 317–320.

Coryell, W. (1978). Intrapatient responses to ECT and tricyclic antidepressants. *American Journal of Psychiatry, 135,* 1108–1110.

Coryell, W. (1982). Hypothalamic-pituitary-adrenal axis abnormality and ECT response. *Psychiatry Research, 6,* 283–292.

Coryell, W., & Zimmerman, M. (1983). The dexamethasone suppression test and ECT outcome: A six-month follow-up. *Biological Psychiatry, 18,* 21–27.

Cronholm, B., & Ottosson, J. O. (1961). Memory functions in endogenous depression: Before and after electroconvulsive therapy. *Archives of General Psychiatry, 5,* 193–199.

Cronholm, B., & Ottosson, J. O. (1963). The experience of memory function after electroconvulsive therapy. *British Journal of Psychiatry, 109,* 251–258.

Daniel, W. F., & Crovitz, H. F. (1982). Recovery of orientation after electroconvulsive therapy. *Acta Psychiatrica Scandinavica, 66,* 421–428.

Daniel, W. F., & Crovitz, H. F. (1983a). Acute memory impairment following electroconvulsive therapy. 1. Effects of electrical stimulus waveform and number of treatments. *Acta Psychiatrica Scandinavica, 67,* 1–7.

Daniel, W. F., & Crovitz, H. F. (1983b). Acute memory impariment following electroconvulsive therapy. 2. Effects of electrode placement. *Acta Psychiatrica Scandinavica, 67,* 57–68.

Deakin, J. F. W., Ferrier, I. N., Crow, T. J., Johnstone, E. C., & Lawler, P. (1983). Effects of ECT on pituitary hormone release: Relationship to seizure, clinical variables and outcome. *British Journal of Psychiatry, 143,* 618–624.

Decina, P., Sackheim, H. A., & Malitz, S. (1983). Prognostic value of serial dexamethasone suppression tests during and following ECT. *Psychopharmacology Bulletin, 19,* 85–87.

Dornbush, R. L., Abrams, R., & Fink, M. (1971). Memory changes after unilateral and bilateral convulsive therapy. *British Journal of Psychiatry, 119,* 75–78.

Ehrensing, R. H., Kastin, A. J., Schalach, D. S., Friesen, H. G., Vargas, J. R., & Schally, A. V. (1974). Affective states and thyrotropin and prolactin responses after repeated injections of TRH in depressed patients. *American Journal of Psychiatry, 131,* 714–718.

d'Elia, G. (1970). Unilateral electroconvulsive therapy. *Acta Psychiatrica Scandinavica,* (Suppl. 215), pp. 1–98.

Elliott, D. L., Linz, D. H., & Kane, J. A. (1982). Electroconvulsive therapy. Pretreatment medical evaluation. *Archives of Internal Medicine, 142,* 979–981.

Ettigi, P. G., & Brown, G. N. (1977). Psychoneuroendocrinology of affective disorder: An overview. *American Journal of Psychiatry, 134,* 493–501.

Extein, I., Pottash, A. L. C., Gold, M. S., Cadet, J., Sweeney, D. R., Davis, R. K., & Martin, D. M. (1980). The thyroid-stimulating hormone response to thyrotropin-releasing hormone in mania and bipolar depression. *Psychiatry Research, 2,* 199–204.

Fink, M. (1979). *Convulsive therapy: theory and practice. New York: Raven Press, pp. 45-53, 87-94, 216-222.*

Fink, M. (1982a). Convlusive therapy: A risk-benefit analysis. Psychopharmacology Bulletin, 18, 110–116.

Fink, M. (1982b). Neuroendocrine aspects of convulsive therapy. In R. Abrams & W. B. Essman (Eds.), *Ilelectroconvulsive therapy* (pp. 187–197). New York: Spectrum Publications.

Fink, M. (1982c). Predictors of outcome in convulsive therapy. *Psychopharmacology Bulletin, 18,* 50–57.

Fink, M., Kahn, R. L., & Green, M. (1958). Experimental studies of the electroshock process. *Diseases of the Nervous System, 19,* 113–118.

Fink, M., & Ottosson, J. O. (1980). A theory of convulsive therapy in endogenous depression: Significance of hypothalamic function. *Psychiatry Research, 2,* 49–61.

Fleminger, J. J., Horne, D. J. de L., Nair, N, P. V., & Nott, P. N. (1970). Differential effect of unilateral and bilateral ECT. *American Journal of Psychiatry, 127,* 430–436.

Frankel, F. H. (1982). Medicolegal and ethical aspects of treatment. In R. Abrams & W. B. Essman (Eds.), *Electroconvulsive therapy* (pp. 245-258). New York: Spectrum Publications.

Fraser, R. M., & Glass, I. B. (1978). Recovery from ECT in elderly patients. *British Journal of Psychiatry, 133,* 524–528.

Fraser, R. M., & Glass, I. B. (1980). Unilateral and bilateral ECT in elderly patients. *Acta Psychiatrica Scandinavica, 62,* 13–31.

Freeman, C. P. L., Basson, J. V., & Crichton, A. (1978). Double blind controlled trial of electroconvulsive therapy (ECT) and simulated ECT in depressive illness. *Lancet, 1,* 738–740.

Freeman, C. P. L., & Kendell, R. E. (1980). ECT: I. Patient's experiences and attitudes. *British Journal of Psychiatry, 137,* 8–16.

Freeman, C. P. L., Weeks, D., & Kendell, R. E. (1980). ECT: II. Patients who complain. *British Journal of Psychiatry, 137,* 17–25.

Fromholt, T. P., Christensen, A., & Stromgren, L. S. (1973). The effects of unilateral and bilateral electroconvulsive therapy on memory. *Acta Psychiatrica Scandinavica, 49,* 466–478.

Gerring, J. P., & Shields, H. M. (1982). The identification and management of patients with a high risk for cardiac arrhythmias during modified ECT. *Journal of Clinical Psychiatry, 43,* 140–143.

Glassman, A. J., Kantor, S. J., & Shostak, M. (1975). Depression, delusions and drug response. *American Journal of Psychiatry, 132,* 7 16–719.

Gold, M. S., Pottash, A. L. C., Extein, I., Martin, D. M., Howard, E., Mueller, E. A. III, & Sweeney, D. R. (1981). The TRH test in the diagnosis of major and minor depression. *Psychoneuroendocrinology, 6,* 159–169.

Gold, M. S., Pottash, A. L. C., Ryan, N., Sweeney, D. R., Davies, R. K., & Martin, D. M. (1980). TRH-induced response in unipolar, bipolar, and secondary depressions: Possible utility in clinical assessment and differential diagnosis. *Psychoneuroendocrinology, 5,* 147–155.

Goldman, H., Gomer, F. E., & Templer, D. I. (1972). Long-term effects of electroconvulsive therapy upon memory and perceptual motor performance. *Journal of Clinical Psychology, 28,* 32–34.

Gomez, J. (1975). Subjective side effects of ECT. *British Journal of Psychiatry, 127,* 609–611.

Gottlieb, G., & Wilson, I. (1965). Cerebral dominance: Temporary disruption of verbal memory by unilateral electroconvulsive shock treatment. *Journal of Comparative and Physiological Psychology, 60,* 368–372.

Gregoire, F., Brauman, H., DeBuck, R., & Corvilain, J. (1977). Hormone release in depressed patients before and after recovery. *Psychoneuroendocrinology, 2,* 303–312.

Grimm, &., & Reichlin, S. (1973). Thyrotropin releasing hormone (TRH): Neurotransmitter regulation of secretion by mouse hypothalamic tissue *in vitro. Endocrinology, 93,* 626–631.

Halliday, A. M., Davison, K., Browne, M. W., & Kreeger, L. C. (1968). A comparison of the effects on depression and memory of bilateral ECT and unilateral ECT to the dominant and nondominant hemisphere. *British Journal of Psychiatry, 114,* 997–1012.

Hargreaves, W. A., Fischer, A., Elashoff, R. M., & Blacker, K. H. (1972). Delayed onset of impairment following electrically induced convulsions. *Acta Psychiatrica Scandinavica, 48,* 69–77.

Haskett, R. J. (1982). Factors affecting outcome after successful electroconvulsive therapy. *Psychopharmacological Bulletin, 18,* 75–78.

Haskett, R. F., & Albala, A. A. (1982). Relevance of neuroendocrine strategies for electroconvulsive therapy research. *Psychopharmacological Bulletin, 18,* 57–62.

Haymaker, W., Anderson, E., & Nauta, W. J. H. (1969). *The hypothalamus.* Springfield, Il: Charles C. Thomas.

Hermoni, M., Lerer, B., Ebstein, R. P., & Belmaker, R. H. (1980). Chronic lithium prevents reserpine induced supersensitivity of adenylate cyclase. *Journal of Pharmacy and Pharmacology, 32,* 510–511.

Hoenig, J., & Chaulk, R. (1977). Delirium associated with lithium therapy and electroconvulsive therapy. *Canadian Medical Association Journal, 116,* 837–838.

Hughes, J., Barraclough, B. M., & Reeve, W. (1981). Are patients shocked by ECT? *Journal of the Royal Society of Medicine, 1981, 74,* 283–285.

Impastato, D. J., & Karlinger, W. (1966). Control of memory impairment in EST by unilateral stimulation of the non-dominant hemisphere. *Diseases of the Nervous System, 27,* 182–188.

Jackson, B. (1978). The effects of unilateral and bilateral ECT on verbal and visual spatial memory. *Journal of Clinical Psychology, 34,* 4–13.

Jefferson, J. W. (1975). A review of the cardiovascular effects and toxicity of tricyclic antidepressants. *Psychosomatic Medicine, 37,* 160–179. Johnstone, E, C., Deakin, J. F. W., Lawler, P., Frith, C. D., Stevens, M., McPherson, K., & Crow, T. J. (1980). The Northwick Park ECT trial. *Lancet, 2,* 1317–1320.

Kahn, R. L., Zarit, S. H., Hilbert, N. M. & Niederehe, G. (1975). Memory complaint and impairment in the aged. *Archives of General Psychiatry, 32,* 1569–1573.

Kalinowsky, L. B. (1945). Organic psychotic syndromes occurring during electric convulsive therapy. *Archives of Neurology and Psychiatry, 53,* 269–273.

Karliner, W., & Wehrheim, H. K. (1965). Maintenance convulsive treatments. *American Journal of Psychiatry, 121,* 113–115.

Kaskey, G. B., Nasr, S., & Meltzer, H. Y. (1980). Drug treatment in delusional depression. *Psychiatry Research, 1,* 267–277.

Kastin, A. J., Ehrensing, R. H., Schalch, D. S., & Anderson, M. S. (1972). Improvement in mental depression with decreased thyrotropin response after administration of thyrotropin-releasing hormone. *Lancet, 2,* 740–742.

Kendell, R. E. (1981). The present status of electroconvulsive therapy. *British Journal of Psychiatry, 139,* 265–283.

Kendler, K. S., & Davis, K. L. (1977). Elevated corticosteroids as a possible cause of abnormal neuroendocrine functions in depressive illness. *Communication in Psychopharmacology, 3,* 183–193.

Kirkegaard, C. (1981). The thyrotropin response to thyrotropin-releasing hormone in endogenous depression. *Psychoneuroendocrinology, 6,* 198–212.

Kirkegaard, C., Bjorum, N., Cohn, D., & Lauridsen, B. U. (1978). Thyrotropin-releasing hormone (TRH) stimulation test in manic-depressive illness. *Archives of General Psychiatry, 35,* 1017–1021.

Kirkegaard, C., Norlem, N., Lauridsen, B. U., Bjorum, N., & Christiansen, C. (1975). Protirelin stimulation test and thyroid function during treatment of depression. *Archives of General Psychiatry, 32,* 1115–1118.

Kirkegaard, C., & Smith, E. (1978). Continuation therapy in endogenous depression controlled by changes in the TRH stimulation test. *Psychological Medicine, 8,* 501–503.

Lancaster, N. P., Steinert, R. R., & Frost, I. (1958). Unilateral electroconvulsive therapy. *Journal of Mental Science, 104,* 221–227.

Lerer, B., & Belmaker, R. H. (1982). Receptors and their mechanism of action of ECT. *Biological Psychiatry, 17,* 497–511.

Linkowski, P., Brauman, H., & Mendelwicz, J. (1981). Thyrotropin response to TRH in unipolar and bipolar affective illness. *Journal of Affective Disorders, 3,* 9–16.

Linnoila, M., Karoum, F., Rosenthal, M., & Potter, W. Z. (1983). Electroconvulsive treatment and lithium carbonate. Their effects on norepinephrine metabolism in patients with primary, major depressions. *ARchives of General Psychiatry, 40,* 677–680.

Loosen, P. T., & Prange, A. J., Jr. (1982). Serum thyrotropin response to thyrotropin-releasing hormone in psychiatric patients: A review. *American Journal of Psychiatry, 139,* 405–416.

Maletzky, B. M. (1978). Seizure duration and clinical effect in electroconvulsive therapy. *Comprehensive Psychiatry, 19,* 541–550.

Mandel, M. R., Madsen, J., Miller, A. L., & Baldessarini, R. J. (1980). Intoxication associated with lithium and ECT. *American Journal of Psychiatry, 137,* 1107–1109.

Marshall, J. R., Kalin, N., & Tariot, A. M. (1980). An organic psychosis associated with electroconvulsive therapy. *Psychiatric Opinion, 17,* 33–39.

McCabe, M. S. (1976). ECT in the treatment of manics: A controlled study. *American Journal of Psychiatry, 133,* 688–691.

McCabe, M. S., & Norris, B. (1977). ECT versus chlorpromazine in mania. *Biological Psychiatry, 12,* 245–254.

Miller, E. (1970). The effect of ECT on memory and learning. *British Journal of Medical Psychology, 43,* 57–62.

Mondimore, F. M., Damlouji, N., Folstein, M. F., & Tune, L. (1983). Post-ECT confusional states associated with elevated serum anticholinergic levels. *American Journal of Psychiatry, 140,* 930–931.

Mowbray, R. M. (1954). Disorientation for age. *Journal of Mental Science, 100,* 749–752.

O'Dea, J. P. K., Gould, D., Hallberg, M., & Weiland, P. G. (1978). Prolactin changes during electroconvulsive therapy. *American Journal of Psychiatry, 135,* 609–611.

Ottosson, J. O. (1960). Experimental studies in the mode of action of electroconvulsive therapy. *Acta Psychiatrica Scandinavica* (Suppl.), *145,* 1–41.

Pandy, G. M., Heinze, W. J., Brown, B. D., & Davis, J. M. (1979). Electroconvulsive shock treatment decreases beta-adrenergic receptor sensitivity in rat brain. *Nature, 280,* 234–235.

Papakostas, Y., Fink, M., Lee, J., Irwin, P., & Johnson, L. (1981). Neuroendocrine measures in psychiatric patients: Course and outcome with ECT. *Psychiatry Research, 4,* 55–64.

Paul, S. M., Extein, I., Calil. H. M., Potter, W. Z., Chodoff, P., & Goodwin, F. K. (1981). Use of ECT with treatment-resistant deprived patients at the National Institute of Mental Health. *American Journal of Psychiatry, 138,* 486–489.

Pettinati, H. M., & Bonner, K. M. (1984). Cognitive functioning in depressed geriatric patients with a history of ECT. *American Journal of Psychiatry, 141,* 49–52.

Pitts, F. N., Jr. (1982). Medical physiology of ECT. In R. Abrams & W. B. Essman (Eds.), *Eletroconvulsive therapy* (pp. 57-89). New York: Spectrum Publications.

Pitts, F. N., Jr., Desmarais, G. M., Stewart, W., & Shaberg, K. (1965). Induction of anesthesia with methohexital and thiopental in electroconvulsive therapy. *New England Journal of Medicine, 273,* 353–360.

Prange, A. J., Wilson, I. C., Lara, P. P., Alltop, L. B., & Breese, G. R. (1972). Effects thyrotropin-releasing hormone in depression. *Lancet, 2,* 999–1002,

Price, T. R. P. (1981). Unilateral electroconvulsive therapy for depression. *New England Journal of Medicine, 304,* 53–55.

Price, T. R. P. (1982a). Short- and long-term cognitive effects of ECT: Part I—Effects on memory. *Psychopharmacology Bulletin, 18,* 81–91.

Price, T. R. P. (1982b). Short-and long-term cognitive effects of ECT: Part II—Effects of nonmemory associated cognitive functions. *Psychopharmacology Bulletin, 18*, 91–101.

Rao, V. A. R., & Coppen, A. (1979). Classification of depression and response to antriptylene therapy. *Psychological Medicine, 9*, 321–325.

Reichert, H., Benjamin, J., Keegan, D., & Majerreson, G. (1976). Bilateral and non-dominant unilateral ECT. I. Therapeutic efficacy. *Canadian Psychiatric Association Journal, 21*, 69–78.

Remick, R. A., & Maurice, W. L. (1978). ECT in pregnancy. *American Journal of Psychiatry, 135*, 761–762.

Sachar, E. J. (1981). Psychobiology of affective disorders. In E. R. Kandel & J. H. Schwartz (Eds.), *Principles of neural science* (pp. 611-619). New York: Elsevier/North-Holland.

Salzman, C. (1982). Electroconvulsive therapy in the elderly patient. Psychiatric *Clinics of North America, 5*, 191–197.

Schou, M. (1980). Pharmacology and toxicity of lithium. In F. Hoffmeister & G. Stille (Eds.), *Psychotropic agents. Part I. Antipsychotics and antidepressants* (pp. 581–589.). New York: Springer-Verlag.

Scovern, A. W., & Kilmann, P. R. (1980). Status of electroconvulsive therapy: Review of outcome literature. *Psychological Bulletin, 87*, 260–303.

Siris, S. G., Glassman, A. H., & Stetner, F. (1982). ECT and psychotropic medication in the treatment of depression and schizophrenia. In R. Abrams & W. B. Essman (Eds.), *Electroconvulsive therapy* (pp. 91-111). New York: Spectrum Publications.

Small, J. G., Kellams, J. J., Milstein, V., & Small, I. F. (1980). Complications with electroconvulsive treatment combined with lithium. *Biological Psychiatry, 15*, 103–112.

Small, J. G., & Small, I. F. (1981). Electroconvulsive therapy update. *Psychopharmacology Bulletin, 17*, 29–42.

Spanis, C. W., & Squire, L. R. (1981). Memory and convulsive stimulation: Effects of stimulus waveform. *American Journal of Psychiatry, 138*, 1177–1181.

Squire, L. R. (1975). A stable impairment in remote memory following electroconvulsive therapy. *Neuropsychologia, 13*, 51–58.

Squire, L. R. (1977). ECT and memory loss. *American Journal of Psychiatry, 134*, 997–1001.

Squire, L. R. (1982). Neuropsychological effects of ECT. In R. Abrams & W. B. Essman (Eds.), *Electroconvulsive therapy* (pp. 169-186). New York: Spectrum Publications.

Squire, L. R., & Chace, P. M. (1975). Memory functions six to nine months after electroconvulsive therapy. *Archives of General Psychiatry, 125*, 490–495.

Squire, L. R., Chace, P. M., & Slater, P. C. (1976). Retrograde amnesia following electroconvulsive therapy. *Nature, 260*, 776–777.

Squire, L. R., & Miller, P. L. (1974). Diminution of anterograde amnesia following electroconvulsive therapy. *British Journal of Psychiatry, 125*, 490–495.

Squire, L. R., Slater, P. C., & Chace, P. M. (1975). Retrograde amnesia: Temporal gradient in very long-term memory following electroconvulsive therapy. *Science, 187*, 77–79.

Squire, L. R., Slater, P. C., & Miller, P. L. (1980). Retrograde amnesia following ECT: Long-term follow-up studies. *Archives of General Psychiatry, 38*, 89–85.

Squire, L. R., Wetzel, C. D., & Slater, P. C. (1978). Anterograde amnesia following ECT: An analysis of the beneficial effects of partial information. *Neuropsychologia. 15,* 339–348.

Squire, L. R., Wetzel, C. D., & Slater, P. C. (1979). Memory complaint after electroconvulsive therapy: Assessment with a new self-rating scale. *Biological Psychiatry, 14,* 791–801.

Stancer, H. C., Quarrington, B., Cookston, B. A., Brown, G. M., Bonkalo, A., & Lyall, W. A. L. (1969). A longitudinal drug study and central amines. *Archives of General Psychiatry, 20,* 290–300.

Sternberg, E. D., & Jarvik, M. E. (1976). Memory functions in depression. *Archives of General Psychiatry, 33,* 219–224.

Stromgren, L. S. (1977). The influence of depression on memory. *Acta Psychiatrica Scandinavica, 56,* 109–128.

Summers, W. K., Robins, E., & Reich, T. (1979). The natural history of acute organic mental syndrome after bilateral electroconvulsive therapy. *Biological Psychiatry, 14,* 905–912.

Taylor, J. R., Tompkins, R., Demers, R., & Anderson, D. (1982). Electroconvulsive therapy and memory dysfunction: Is there evidence for prolonged defects? *Biological Psychiatry, 17,* 1169–1193.

Taylor, M. A. (1982). Indications for electroconvulsive therapy. In R. Abrams & W. B. Essman (Eds.), *Electroconvulsive therapy* (pp. 7-39). New York: Spectrum Publications.

Thomann, P., & Hess, R. (1980). Toxicology of antidepressant drugs. In F. Hoffmeister & G. Stille (Eds.), *Psychotropic agents. Part I. Antipsychotics and antidepressants* (pp. 527–549.). New York: Springer-Verlag.

Thomas, J., & Reddy, B. (1982). The treatment of mania. A retrospective evaluation of the effects of ECT, chlorpromazine, and lithium. *Journal of Affective Disorders, 4,* 85–92-

Valentine, M., Keddie, K. M. G., & Dunne, D. (1968). A comparison of techniques in electroconvulsive therapy. *British Journal of Psychiatry, 114,* 989–996.

Weaver, L. A., Ives, J. O., Williams, R., & Nies, A. (1977). A comparison on standard alternating current and low energy brief-pulse electrotherapy. *Biological Psychiatry, 12,* 525–543.

Weeks, D., Freeman, C. P. L., & Kendell, R. E. (1980). ECT: III. Enduring cognitive deficits. *British Journal of Psychiatry, A review of the literature. American Journal of Psychiatry, 137,* 26–37.

Weiner, R. D., Whanger, A. D., Erwin, C., & Wilson, W. P. (1980). Prolonged confusional state and EEG seizure activity following concurrent ECT and lithium use. *American Journal of Psychiatry, 137,* 1452–1453.

Welch, C. A. (1982). The relative efficacy of unrelated nondominant and bilateral stimulation. *Psychopharmacology Bulletin, 18,* 68–70.

Wexler, B. E. (1980). Cerebral laterality and psychiatry, 137, 279–291.

Wilson, I., & Gottlieb, G. (1967). Unilateral electroconvulsive shock therapy. *Diseases of the Nervous System, 28,* 541–545.

Zubin, J. (1948). Memory functioning in patients treated with electric shock therapy. *Journal of Personality, 17,* 33–41.

7

Symbolic Interactionism: A Framework for Interventions with the Hospitalized Suicidal Patient

Marian Fiske
Marsha D. Snyder

Suicide, with its threat pervasive and ever-present in the hospital milieu, has been characterized as the "cardiac arrest of the psychiatric unit." Its rate is 30% higher than in the general population (Farberow, 1981). Suicide challenges and mocks the staff's dedication to the preservation and enhancement of life. Interest in the subject has greatly intensified over the past two decades with articles, books, and studies devoted to the search for the who's, why's, and how's of this major health problem. Scales, questionnaires, and checklists appear in a quest for the perfect instrument to identify clearly the suicidally intent person, but the self-destruction continues.

Responding to this serious concern, the authors will briefly review current information about suicide and the hospitalized psychiatric patient, discuss the perspective of symbolic interactionism and its application to the care and treatment of the suicidal patient, and finally examine impediments that may preclude a successful outcome regardless of the preventative measures.

SUICIDE AND THE HOSPITALIZED PSYCHIATRIC PATIENT

It is not surprising that suicides occur more commonly in psychiatric facilities than in other surroundings because the most disturbed patients seek inpatient care (Farberow, 1981), Many practitioners provide outpatient treatment for as long as possible to those with suicidal ideation. Once a suicide attempt is initiated or seems imminent, hospitalization becomes the choice of treatment. The community at large, as well as psychiatric professionals, expect the staff on psychiatric units to intervene in the suicide process and convince the patient that there is hope and life is worth living. Thus, the hospital setting is used primarily to provide a safe environment as well as minimize opportunities for patients to harm themselves (Litman & Farberow, 1966).

A number of risk factors have been associated with suicide among psychiatric patients. History of previous attempt has been well-documented (Beisser & Blanchette, 1961; Roy, 1982). Roy (1982) added the factors of previous psychiatric hospitalizations or treatment or both, and also found suicide more common among the unmarried, the unemployed, and the person living alone. In this population, men were more likely to kill themselves than women. In addition, the men were significantly younger (Beisser & Blanchette, 1961; Roy, 1982). Men also used more lethal methods to complete the act (Roy, 1982). Two separate studies found that of those who commit suicide, approximately 60% were male and 40% were female (Beisser & Blanchette, 1961; Roy, 1982).

The clinical features of depression are frequently tied to suicidal behavior in psychiatric patients (Beisser & Blanchette, 1961; Farberow, 1981; Roose et al., 1983; Roy, 1982; Sletten et al., 1972). When depressive symptoms are accompanied by hostile, irritable, withdrawn, isolative behavior, a patient's self-destructive impulses become heightened (Farberow, 1981). If delusions are present, suicide risk increases (Roose, et al., 1983). A chronic picture of these symptoms matched with disorganized thought processes leads to schizophrenia as the second most common diagnosis among psychiatric patients who commit suicide (Beisser & Blanchette, 1961; Farberow, 1981; Roy, 1982; Sletten et al., 1972). This latter group often chooses the most lethal methods for suicide.

A profile of the hospitalized suicidal patient emerges from the previously mentioned data. If male, this individual will probably be younger than his female counterpart. More than likely he or she will be unemployed, unmarried, living alone, and have a clinical picture of depression with psychotic features. In addition, this patient will probably have a history of either previous psychiatric hospitalization, or treatment, or both and have made suicide attempts in the past.

SYMBOLIC INTERACTIONISM: ITS APPLICATION TO CARE AND TREATMENT OF THE SUICIDAL PATIENT

Symbolic interactionism is a perspective in social psychology particularly relevant to the care of the suicidal patient. It focuses on the nature of interaction and sees human beings as active, emerging, and changing through this process.

Symbolic interactionism encompasses the following premises:*

1. Human beings act toward the objects in their world on the basis of the meaning these objects have for them.
2. These meanings are derived through social interaction with other people, using both verbal and nonverbal language.
3. People modify and handle the meanings of objects in their world through an interpretive process.

The objects in a person's world comprise all those things that he or she points out, recognizes, and acknowledges. This includes everything from a chair, a book, and a friend, to abstract ideas of freedom, justice, and compassion. The nature of any object consists of the meaning it has for the person referring to it. Meaning sets the way a person sees and acts toward the things in his or her environment; a door will then be a different object to a city home owner, then to either an antique dealer or a psychiatric inpatient. An overwhelming task for one person becomes a challenge for the next (Blumer, 1969).

Each person learns the meaning of objects through observing the way other people he or she encounters identify and use them. Meanings are social products created by people interacting with one another and change as use of objects change. So a chest becomes something to sit on, a place to store things in, or it can become a valuable collector's item (Charon, 1979).

Behavior, however, does not result from a direct application of these learned meanings. First, people carry out an internal dialogue with themselves, indicating those things in their world to which they respond. They then modify and transform these meanings in light of the present situation and past experiences. Through this process of self-communication, new lines of action are developed based on these modified meanings (Blumer, 1969). For example, an anxious young woman waiting in a doctor's anteroom begins to relax as she notes the comfortable furniture, soft lighting, and warm concerned manners of the receptionist. She says to herself, "This office seems calm and efficient. It reminds me of my living room, where I always feel safe. I think I will be helped here." Suddenly, a scream pierces the air and a nurse hurries by carrying a large syringe. The woman tenses and tells herself, "Somebody is being hurt. Needles are painful. A nurse rushing by means something has gone wrong. That's how it was when Uncle John died. This is not a good place. I won't stay." She gets up and leaves. Through self dialogue, the young woman transforms the doctor's office from a place of help and safety to a site of potential harm.

This inner conversation results because each person has a self and can be an

---

*Blumer, H. (1969). *Symbolic interactionism: Perspective and method* (pp. 1–16). Englewood Cliffs, NJ: Prentice-Hall. © 1969. Reprinted by permission of Prentice-Hall, Inc., Englewood Cliffs, N.J.

object of his or her own action. The way people define the self is the way individuals act toward themselves. As with all objects, this definition arises out of interaction with others: People come to view and understand themselves from the way others point out and define them (Blumer, 1969). For example, from her immediate family, Jane learns and begins to see herself as ''a girl, cute and pretty, smarter than her brother John, and the image of Aunt Margaret, the bank president.''**

The development of self as object progresses from the child's assumption of one significant other's perception at a time, to the adult's incorporation of all significant others' perceptions as one ''generalized other'' (Mead, 1934). This internalized set of attitudes of others is termed the ''me'' by Mead while the adjusted response to these attitudes denotes the ''I'' or subjective self. Through the internal dialogue between the ''I'' and ''me,'' an individual controls, judges, and plans actions toward the objects encountered in his or her world (Blumer, 1969; Charon, 1979).

Through this perspective, a person's social world consists only of objects that are known and recognized. Communication occurs when meanings are shared, agreed upon, and negotiated. New meanings, including the definition of self and resulting new lines of action, develop through an interactive interpretive process with others.

In applying this perspective to the care of hospitalized suicidal patients, the nurse must enter the social world of these individuals and learn the meaning and consequences of their particular rules and formulas. When the nurse understands the meanings of the patients' world, she or he can help them to modify and alter their restricted view of alternative solutions to problems.

ASSESSING RISK: THE LANGUAGE OF SUICIDE

All of the aforementioned demographic, social, and psychological factors provide a working framework for the assessment of the suicidal individual. However, if the patient's unique meanings are overlooked or ignored, important clues may be lost. The following example illustrates this process:

Jane, a young nurse, reported she had just admitted a 50-year-old depressed, agitated woman. All the right questions—including those pertaining to self-harm—had been asked. The patient denied any such ideas. However, Jane found one aspect of the interaction quite puzzling. Several pieces of valuable jewelry had been brought in by the patient who stated she always liked to have them with her when traveling. Jane informed her that

**Charon, J. M. (1979). *Symbolic interactionism: An introduction, an interpretation, an integration* (pp. 38–39, 63–85). Englewood Cliffs, NJ: Prentice-Hall. © 1979. Adapted by permission of Prentice-Hall, Inc., Englewood Cliffs, N.J.

for safety's sake, the jewelry should be put in the vault since she was now hospitalized and would not be traveling; reluctantly, the patient agreed. Since Jane did not equate hospitalization as travel, she labeled the patient delusional. On hearing this report, the supervisor suggested that she discuss traveling and its meaning with the patient. When the patient began to ramble about peaceful islands with blue skies and sandy beaches, Jane thought she was referring to some Caribbean vacation spot. Slowly she realized the patient was fantasizing about another and better world. Finally, the patient disclosed her well-thought-out suicide plan.

Although each person's definitions and resulting behavior are highly individualistic, several patterns exist that are characteristic of many people comtemplating suicide. The first is an increasing expression of agitation, anguish, fear, and hopelessness. Shneidman (1976) uses the word "perturbation" to describe this state. He defines it as "how upset, disturbed, and discouraged the person is." The second pattern relates to the narrowing focus in the person's perspective of his or her situation until suicide seems the only reasonable solution to end the pain. Anguish and helplessness become the person's whole world with all emotional energies directed toward the unbearable pain and its resolution. All external stimuli are interpreted in light of these anguished perceptions. An awareness of surroundings diminishes except in relation to the self, and becomes magnified and distorted. The patient interprets and defines all interactions based on this heightened and disturbed self-consciousness. Thus, a busy staff member passing by with only a nod of recognition, may be defined as rejecting by the suicidal patient. These patterns of anguish and disturbed perception are graphically illustrated by Savage (1979) in recounting her personal struggle with suicide.

I had gone to see my medical doctor about a kidney infection, and although he did everything possible, I came away with the feeling that he didn't care. On that day, too, I had seen my therapist, and, as he had failed to do something I expected him to do, I felt that he didn't care either . . . .

I was permeated with a profound sense of degradation, of helplessness and hopelessness, of being boxed into a situation from which there was no exit. My life was a trap, and I was running around inside it in meaningless patterns that didn't go anywhere or produce anything, and all around me was the twilight of despair that grew ever deeper and thicker, with not even the suggestion of a promise that there could ever be a dawn.

Another patient, after recovering from a serious suicide attempt—the ingestion of 30 seconal—described the process as "walking into a steadily darkening cornicopia." As the walls of the cornicopia pressed in on her—a metaphor for what she saw as an intolerable life situation—she knew she would have to die when she reached the tip of this narrowing tunnel.

Because such feelings are so intense to the patient, he or she often assumes this state to be readily apparent to others. The patient feels as if the inner dialogue were on a loudspeaker system with everyone listening. While some patients express their anguish directly, through speaking of fears and hopelessness, others respond more silently through agitation, pacing, isolation, or withdrawal. Still others manifest their despair in delusions and hallucinations. Although increased anguish and constriction of perception seem to be easily recognized signs of the potentially suicidal patient, in fact, only minimal changes of behavior can result. Busy unit staff may easily overlook these behavioral signs. While the patient feels he or she is sending up rockets of distress, staff may see only the wave of a finger. This situation demonstrates why the suicidal patient may go unrecognized.

Most psychiatric nurses know the cardinal rules for assessing suicidal ideation: talk to the patient directly, find out if he or she has a plan, how lethal it is and what the likelihood is of it being carried out. Ask if the patient has felt this way or tried to commit suicide before. On a busy inpatient unit, however, none of these questions may be asked if the patient's distress signals go unnoticed. For patients admitted because of serious suicide threats and attempts, which is a major reason for psychiatric hospitalization, the ongoing assessment can become routine and a small increase in despair can go unrecognized. The process of staff recognition of this change becomes even more problematic for patients who develop suicidal behavior while hospitalized. The world of the staff may be wide and varied but the patient's world is dark and narrow. Staff members have difficulty in looking through the restricted, self-centered, hypersensitive lens of the patient for an extended period.

Anne, a 65 year old widow, came to the hospital severely depressed and despondent. Since her husband's death a year earlier, her depression and inability to function steadily increased. At first, she refused to participate in unit activities, sitting silent and forlorn in the day room. The nursing staff assisted her with dressing and eating, sitting with her for extended periods, while attempting to build a sense of security and trust. They encouraged her to interact with others. When Anne's daughter and son-in-law reported she told them that the nursing staff tortured and placed her in chains, they were astonished. When the staff approached her, she repeated the charge. Rationalizing that one should not dwell on a patient's delusions, the staff proceeded with their previous plan, ignoring her allegations. Anne appeared to improve, however, talking with other patients, participating in occupational therapy, and expressing a desire to go out on pass, Everyone agreed with the idea, giving her an overnight pass to be with her daughter. While on her leave, the staff heard that Anne had drunk corrosive fluid. Her final words as she lay dying were ''At last I am at peace. This will end the torture I have endured.'' It was clear that nothing had changed while Anne was hospitalized. She had simply stopped talking about her anguish, perhaps believing that staff did not want to hear about the delusional charges she had made against them.

PROBLEMS IN ASSESSMENT: INCONGRUITY OF MEANINGS

This illustration leads to another area of difficulty in caring for and assessing the suicidal patient—the clash of definitions. The staff appear dedicated to the definition that help and hope exist even for the most disturbed and nonfunctional patient. They believe their role is to help patients find ways to cope with their difficulties and improve their life situations. Yet the suicidal patient's definition that there is no hope and only one solution—death—defies this belief. If the patient appears to reject all offers of help, staff may react with anger, withdraw, and stop listening to the coded cry for help. Although this more direct clash of definitions creates conflict, the most difficult problem for staff to deal with is a more subtle message of manipulation by the patient who threatens suicide.

In a study of 200 patients hospitalized for attempted suicide, Beck et al., (1979) found 56% wished to escape from an intolerable life situation, 13% made the attempt in the hope of producing some change in their significant others or their environment, and 31% reported a combination of desire for surcease and an attempt to manipulate. This manipulative aspect may be expressed as a plea for unquestioning love, affection, and approval from significant others; a demand for recognition of the patient's feelings of helplessness; or a desire for revenge and an attempt to blame others for the person's present plight.

Although these messages are usually directed toward meaningful others outside the hospital, they can be aimed at care givers trying to help the patient. This behavior may alienate and anger staff, who withdraw and often label the patient as "manipulative and not really suicidal." Although every human being frequently uses various forms of manipulation throughout life, the label takes on a particularly pejorative meaning in the psychiatric setting: it denotes callow and demanding use and control of others for childish, self-centered ends. No psychiatric staff nurse wants to get caught in such a web and be told by fellow staff "You're being manipulated by that patient." In some cases, sophisticated practicing nurses and graduate students have been immobilized by this particular clash of definitions.

Certainly, there are patients who repeatedly threaten suicide whenever they do not get what they perceive as the right response in interactions with others. Rather than just being labeled manipulative, however, this patient needs help in sorting out the meaning underlying this threat. Ipso facto, the nurse must understand these meanings before trying to help the patient make changes. If neither action occurs, the clash of definitions continues.

Finally, even the suicidal patient's message of death can be confusing. For many people, suicide does not appear to mean the end of life but rather a new beginning. They often indicate directly or indirectly that they do not perceive a difference between death and nonterminal escape, even to witnessing the reaction of others to their death. This misperception was illustrated in the first example when the newly admitted patient talked about taking her jewelry on her trip to a better world. In this instance the supervisor, an experienced psychiatric nurse, immediately recognized the suicide potential, confirmed by further interaction between the patient and the young nurse. All too often the label "delusional" or "psychotic" is quickly applied to this kind of definition without further exploration of the patient's meaning. This process is particularly important with the depressed delusional patient and the psychotic schizophrenic since these patients more often successfully kill themselves while hospitalized. Their communication of despair is probably so coded and distorted it goes unrecognized.

ENTERING THE SUICIDAL PATIENT'S WORLD

It is crucial for the nurse to enter the suicidal patient's world and learn the meaning of symbols used to govern his or her behavior. Two prerequisites mediate the effectiveness of this process. First, nurses must carefully identify the rules and prescriptions used to organize and direct their own behavior. This becomes no easy task since most people go about their daily lives quite automatically without questioning or focusing on the underlying belief systems governing their behavior. Shared meaning is often assumed when actually no such agreement occurs. The clash of definitions previously discussed is one of the results of this erroneous assumption. Even more serious is the lack of recognition that such a clash exists. Definitions are simply superimposed on the patient's world. As a result, it is difficult to identify the suicidal patient through statistical methods and descriptions. The suicidal patient who doesn't fit these stereotypes may go unrecognized and no attempt is made to explore and evaluate this patient's world of misery.

A study measuring the reliability with which mental health professionals assess suicidal risk was carried out using a series of videotaped patient interviews (Kaplan et al., 1982). The investigators based suicide risk predominately on two clinical observations: the severity of past suicidal history and "imminence of suicidal feelings". During the study, one of the interviewees killed herself several weeks after discharge. This 64-year-old woman with no previous suicide attempts, but multiple hospitalizations for chronic schizophrenia, had been uniformly rated as low risk. The day before her death she sought help at another hospital, and was again considered nonsuicidal. Apparently, the patient failed to fit the professional mold for suicide potential and the staff failed to crack her code of despair.

Consistent interaction between the nurse and the patient constitutes the second prerequisite for successful entry into the suicidal patient's world. Most people are reluctant to reveal their innermost thoughts and beliefs to others. Only after the nurse is perceived as someone interested, concerned, and willing to listen to explanations and definitions quite different from his or her own, will patients begin to reveal the true parameters of their world. Patients are often aware that the way they see their situation appears quite different from others. Fearful of derision or rejection, they code their definitions with oblique, indirect statements. Only with persistence can shared meanings be worked out between nurse and patient. Unfortunately, the time necessary for this process is difficult to arrange on busy inpatient units. In fact, it has been the authors' experience that patients designated as potentially suicidal are often assigned to less-experienced and sometimes nonprofessional staff to carry out the routine of "suicide precautions." These precautions constitute the plan of graded observations from constant to hourly, and the limitation of access to potentially harmful articles, depending on the patient's condition. They are used by all psychiatric units to protect the patient from self-destructive impulses. Since the suicidal patient is the psychiatric equivalent of the medical intensive care patient, this kind of assignment becomes hard to justify.

Just as the intensive care patient requires the greatest nursing expertise, so does the suicidal patient. Both quality care and a higher ratio of nurses per patient are needed. For the vital consistency required by suicidal patients, it is helpful to limit the number of nurses involved, and to have one primary coordinator of care. Thus, the nurse functions as a major participant in determining and carrying out the observations and interactions required by the precaution procedure. When continual observation is necessary, a limited number of other staff members are involved to avoid subjecting the patient to a constant stream of confusing interactions.

DEVELOPING SHARED DEFINITIONS AS THE BASIS FOR NURSING CARE

Under the symbolic interactionist framework, the goal of care is to help patients expand and change the narrow definitions of their self and world. The plan starts with the development of shared meanings between the nurse and patient concerning the patient's present situation. Opportunities are then provided for the patient to expand and try out new definitions in interacting with others in the unit milieu. This process is not one-sided, directed by the primary nurse, but an ongoing interactive one between the nurse and patient. Contracting is a technique promoting this approach. Contracts may cover a wide range of treatment issues from initial assessment of suicide risk, to ongoing evaluation of suicidal potential and participation in treatment modalities.

In such situations, Drye et al. (1973) have found use of the no-suicide contract particularly effective. Under this method, the patient states, without qualification in terms of a decision rather than a promise or agreement with the evaluator how long he or she is willing to stay alive.

In some settings, not only are no-suicide decisions contracted, but also each goal in the treatment process. In this way, the patient fully participates in setting up contract criteria. Mutual understanding of definitions is essential between nurse and patient. This mutuality promotes fulfillment of expectations and follows with a positive experience for both parties. Inferences or approximate definitions weaken the contract and allow the patient to misinterpret expectations. If the nurse uses the contract as a means to manipulate or control behavior, the process is doomed for failure. Very few patients, if given definitions of control and manipulation implicit in such a contract, would agree to its terms. When mutuality is ignored, disharmony and mistrust enter into the nurse–patient relationship. The patient may view the relationship with anger and resentment. The feeling that the nurse does not care may ensue, "She doesn't care if I live or die . . . . I should die." The nurse, in turn, may mislabel the patient and react inappropriately. Through the processes of supervision and self-examination, practitioners must note when nonmutuality of terms occurs. Once lack of mutuality is recognized, both parties should begin renegotiation of terms. The process of contracting forces mutuality of goals to the forefront.

A contract, however, is not a stagnant agreement or document, but rather a process that evolves. As definitions change, so must the contract. If it is to be effective, the document must be reviewed frequently. Contracting therefore, ensures that communication lines with the suicidal patient are kept open. Open communication lines can save a life as well as decrease frustration and conflict, thus encouraging positive feelings by all involved. The use of a contract between nurse and patient encourages the patient to form mutual relationships. It serves as an important learning task for many patients with limited collaborative experience in previous relationships.

In an experiential study of inpatient treatment of suicidal patients, feelings of impotency and powerlessness were found to be significant characteristics of patienthood (Reynolds & Farberow, 1976). The mutuality of the primary nurse–patient relationship and the collaborative decision-making of contracting, provide an experiential arena for redefining negative characteristics into the more positive attributes of competency and mastery. The procedure of suicide precautions becomes the matrix in which this process takes place. Instead of a tedious, mandated routine, these precautions become a dynamic dialogue between the patient and nurse. Even here, divergent definitions may impede the process. Concerns about patient safety and the legal ramifications of an error in judgment regarding the suicidal patient may lead to overly cautious restrictions on the patient's movement toward independence and self-care.

In the past, the courts assumed that if patients were known to be suicidal, the hospital had full responsibility for keeping them alive. Liability was presumed, no matter what the circumstances, if patients killed or injured themselves (Farberow, 1981). Now the courts recognize that there must be a balance between restrictions necessary to avoid the dangers of suicide, and freedom for patients to assume responsibility for their own behavior. It is generally accepted that liability for an error in judgment will occur only if there is clear evidence of negligence or malpractice (Reis, 1984). Nevertheless, few inpatient units have escaped legal challenges to this concept in our litigious society. Most front-line nurses are well aware of the exceptional risks involved in caring for high risk patients. The dark shadow of potential legal action only increases the anxiety of the nurse already confronting the life-and-death challenge of the suicidal patient.

OTHER TREATMENT MODALITIES

Thus far, interaction between the nurse and patient has been stressed. This approach, however, in no way precludes other treatment modalities such as medication and electroconvulsive therapy (ECT). Effective biological treatment can help expand the patient's ability to contemplate alternatives as symptoms are controlled or alleviated. Here again definitions may effect the treatment process. If medication and ECT use are not understood by the patient, he or she may refuse these treatments, or in the case of medication, prematurely discontinue its use after discharge. By administering and monitoring medicines and preparing patients for ECT, the nurse supplies knowledge about efficacy of these treatments. If the nurse does not know how or why they work, or is ambivalent about their use, the patient will quickly perceive this. Undue anxiety and subsequent loss of an effective therapeutic tool may result.

Despite this variety of treatment modalities, care of the suicidal patient is often difficult and frustrating. New and more positive definitions of self evolve slowly and painfully for the patient, and the process is often marked by ambivalence and resistance. He or she can repeatedly slip into the tunnel vision of self-destruction as the only solution. Much support and encouragement are needed from the nurse even though she may encounter help-rejecting behavior from the patient in this process.

OVERCOMING OBSTACLES TO THE CONTINUITY OF CARE

As noted, the suicidal patient often has a long history of social and psychological difficulties. More than short-term treatment is required to deal with these problems. Studies have shown that the three months following hospitalization becomes the period of highest risk for suicide, and thus, consistent follow-up care is critical for prevention (Farberow, 1981; Roy, 1982). Unfortunately, present day health care economics mitigate against this continuity of care. In an effort to cut down costs of health insurance premiums in the private sector, benefit limitations, deductables, and co-payments have been introduced. Psychiatric services have been particularly hard hit because of the low value placed on mental health benefits. In the public sector, cutbacks have taken place both at the federal and state level (Sharfstein & Patterson, 1983). Ironically, outpatient services have suffered the most. Although hospitalization is available in both sectors, it may be limited to a specific number of days. In outpatient treatment, payment by insurers can be minimal or nonexistent. Community mental health centers have been most affected by the cutbacks in public funds. As a result, the seriously disturbed patient rotates back and forth between public and private hospitals and emergency rooms, with each request for help becoming a new encounter. Continuity is lost in the interactional helping process of developing shared meanings and treatment goals between care giver and patient. Yet, it can be maintained if the patient returns to the same inpatient unit under the care of the same primary nurse or treatment team. All the benefits of a mutually developed consistent relationship can result.

Louise, a middle aged, single clerical worker, entered the inpatient unit five years ago with severe depression and threatening suicide. Hostile and negative, she refused to contract or participate in treatment planning with her primary nurse. Placed on antidepressants, she became less depressed, but at discharge, still refused to participate in unit activities. Fortunate to have insurance that covered outpatient-care by a psychiatrist, she experienced a stormy treatment course. Repeatedly, she returned to thoughts of self-destruction, resulting in hospitalization. Each time she entered the same unit with the same primary nurse. Gradually, she began to modify her negative definitions of herself and her life situation, testing them out in interactions with her primary nurse. She participated in contract decisions regarding self-harm and mutually developed treatment goals. Her social network expanded while she worked regularly and maintained good personal care. The primary nurse and psychiatrist are guardedly optimistic that Louise can eventually eliminate self-destruction as a viable solution to life difficulties.

SUMMARY

Suicidal thoughts, threats, and acts confront the nurse daily in interactions with patients on the inpatient psychiatric unit. No fool-proof method exists that can predict which patients will actually kill themselves. Although statistical and demographic data can provide a framework for the identification process, successful treatment can be achieved only through understanding the meanings and definitions determining the suicidal patient's world. To accomplish this objective, the symbolic interactionist framework has particular relevance. Through the use of primary nursing and contracting, shared meanings and treatment goals can be developed by the nurse and patient. Because suicidal inpatients usually have a history of long-standing, social–psychological problems, continuity in follow-up is important, although present economic sanctions have impeded the process. However, if the patient returns to the same facility with the same primary nurse, continuity of care can be accomplished.

REFERENCES

Beck, A. T., Rush, A. J., Shaw, B. F., & Emery, G. (1979). *Cognitive therapy of depression*. (pp. 211–213). New York: Guilford Press.

Beisser, A. R. & Blanchette, J. E. (1961). A study of suicides in a mental hospital. *Diseases of the Nervous System, 22*, (7), 365–369.

Blumer, H. (1969). *Symbolic interaction: Perspective and method* (pp. 1–16). Englewood Cliffs, NJ: Prentice-Hall.

Charon, J. M. (1979). *Symbolic interactionism: An introduction, an interpretation, an integration* (pp. 63–100). Englewood Cliffs, NJ: Prentice-Hall.

Drye, R. C., Goulding, R. L., & Goulding, M. E. (1973). No-suicide decisions: Patient monitoring of suicidal risk. *American Journal of Psychiatry, 130,* (2), 171–174.

Farberow, N. L. (1981). Suicide prevention in the hospital. *Hospital Community Psychiatry, 32,* 99–103.

Kaplan, R. D., Kottler, D. B., & Frances, A. J. (1982). Reliability and rationality in the prediction of suicide. *Hospital and Community Psychiatry, 33,* 212–215.

Litman, R. E., & Farberow, N. L. (1967). The hospital's obligation toward suicide-prone patients. *Hospitals, 40,* (12), pp. 64–68.

Mead, G. H. (1934). *Mind, self and society* (pp. 135–178). Chicago: University of Chicago Press.

Reis, E. B. (1984). *Mental health and the law.* (pp. 217–224). Rockville, MD: Aspen Systems.

Reynolds, D. K., & Farberow, N. L. (1976). *Suicide inside and out* (pp. 167–171). Berkely: University of California Press.

Roose, S. P., Glassman, A. H., Walsh, B. T., Wodring, S., & Vital-Herne, J. (1983). Depression, delusions, and suicide. *American Journal of Psychiatry, 140,* (9), 1159–1162.

Roy, A. (1982). Risk factors for suicide in psychiatric patients. *Archives of General Psychiatry, 39,* (9), 1089–1095.

Savage, M. (1979). *Addicated to suicide: A woman struggling to live* (pp. 69–78). Cambridge, MA: Schenkman Publishing.

Sharfstein, S. S. & Patterson, D. Y. (1983). The growing crisis in access to mental health services for middle class families. *Hospital and Community Psychiatry, 34,* 1009–1014.

Shneidman, E. S. A psychological theory of suicide. *Psychiatric Annals, 6,* (11), 51–66.

Sletten, I. W., Brown, M. L., Evenson, R. C. & Altman, H. (1972). Suicide in mental hospital patients. *Diseases of the Nervous System, 5,* 328–334.

8

A Practical Guide to Outpatient Differential Therapeutics

Katherine Y. Sasaki

The psychiatric nurse in the out-patient setting practices within a wide spectrum of ambulatory care facilities ranging from partial hospitalization programs, to community mental health centers, to out-patient departments of hospitals. Although the specific role may vary from facility to facility, several nurse-practice treatment modalities will remain common across differing out-patient settings. In these ambulatory care settings, the psychiatric nurse immediately encounters patient case demands for which his or her holistic clinical orientation is particularly well-suited. The out-patient setting is that much closer to patients' usual living situation and hence the therapeutic contact interfaces more intimately with families, jobs, community and friends, and with the patients' responsibility for their own health care (including medications) and for their overall physical well-being. The psychiatric nurses' often extensive contact with patients, whether it be in group or family therapy, in casual, brief encounters several times a day, or in a patient-teaching session on medications, allows a field of observations of everyday behavior that can be the basis upon which to generate an accurate and comprehensive treatment plan.

Working within this framework, the nurse clinician may involve both professional and "natural" or lay-helping networks. She or he considers patients in the entirety of their living context, careful not to plan treatment that disrupts already established therapeutic activities. The nurse recognizes biological ex-

NURSING INTERVENTIONS IN DEPRESSION   Copyright © 1985 by Grune & Stratton, Inc.

Fig. 8-1. The process of differential therapeutics.

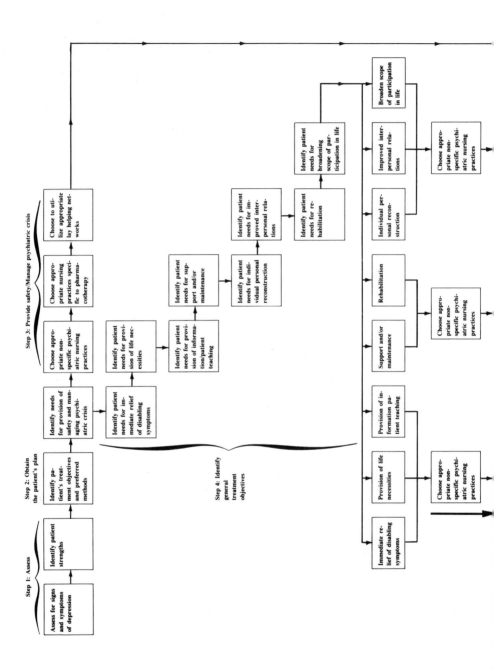

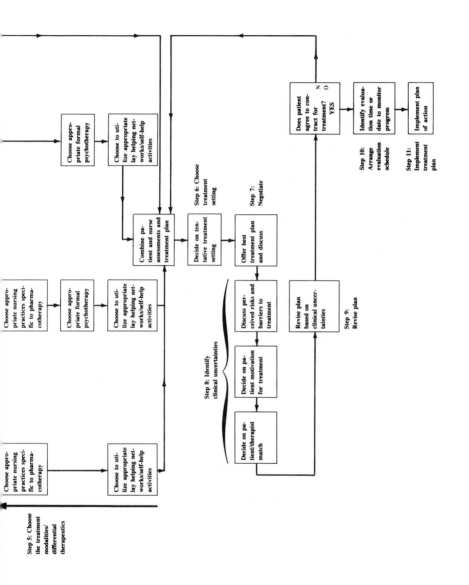

Step 5: Choose the treatment modalities/differential therapeutics

Choose appropriate nursing practices specific to pharmacotherapy

Choose appropriate nursing practices specific to pharmacotherapy

Choose appropriate formal psychotherapy

Choose appropriate formal psychotherapy

Choose to utilize appropriate lay helping networks/self-help activities

Choose to utilize appropriate lay helping networks/self-help activities

Choose to utilize appropriate lay helping networks/self-help activities

Choose to utilize appropriate lay helping networks/self-help activities

Combine patient and nurse assessments and treatment plan

Step 6: Choose treatment setting

Decide on tentative treatment setting

Step 7: Negotiate

Offer best treatment plan and discuss

Step 8: Identify clinical uncertainties

Decide on patient/therapist match

Decide on patient motivation for treatment

Discuss perceived risks and barriers to treatment

Step 9: Revise plan

Revise plan based on clinical uncertainties

Does patient agree to contract for treatment? NO / YES

Step 10: Arrange evaluation schedule

Identify evaluation time or date to monitor progress

Step 11: Implement treatment plan

Implement plan of action

127

pressions of psychopathology that always require monitoring, if not more active intervention. In the process of alleviating dysfunctional behaviors, the scope of such a comprehensive practice leads to creativity in intervention with maximum utilization of patient strengths. This is the challenge for the psychiatric nurse in treating depressed patients on an out-patient basis.

Activating a treatment plan is preceded by a complex, decision-making process based upon accurate assessment of patient needs. This decision-making process, termed *differential therapeutics,* is "a process by which a clinician and patient together choose the most appropriate treatment from among possible alternatives" (Frances & Clarkin, 1981a). This is a formidable task requiring (1) expertise in assessing psychological, interpersonal and social, and biological levels of patient needs; (2) a logical approach to systematically building a treatment plan, exercising an ability to process all pertinent variables in arriving at a sound clinical judgment; (3) a large repetoire of knowledge of and/or expertise in existing treatment modalities with awareness of their comparative efficacies; and (4) a practical and realistic approach to create plans a given patient can accept and engage in.

Weinstein and Fineberg (1980) point out "that good decisions in medicine, although full of clinical uncertainties, is an art which can be learned and perfected through a system based on rational principles." The state of the art of differential therapeutics in psychiatry is as yet young and unrefined. This is demonstrated in the American Psychiatric Association's *Manual of Psychiatric Peer Review* that essentially reveals that many treatments are potentially appropriate for almost every DSM-III diagnosis (Frances & Clarkin, 1981a). Yet psychiatric nurse-clinicians do make treatment decisions every day in the clinical arena with the underlying assumption that choice of treatment modality is significant and relevant to outcome. But upon what data is a decision based, and by what method and justifications? Given the problems of a depressed patient in an out-patient setting, utilizing elements of a decision–analytic approach, a practical guide to the nurse–patient process of differential therapeutics, will be described. This guide, presented in Figure 8-1, will be applicable to all out-patient settings and can be utilized at many points in a given patient's treatment course. The outlined nursing interventions (in Tables 8-1 through 8-9) are of a general nature so as to accommodate the further elaboration of individualized treatment plans. The guide is in the format of a flow chart to suggest a logical, prioritized approach to the complete process of differential therapeutics. Each major step will be addressed in detail.

STEP 1.   ASSESS

In this preliminary step, data on the patient is gathered from a variety of sources; e.g., the patient, physician, family, patient records, and other healthcare providers. Signs and symptoms of depression are assessed.* The assessment must be based upon a holistic model such as the Integrated Model of Depression (Akiskal & McKinney, 1975). This model views occurrence of primary depression as the result of an interplay of experiential, chemical, and behavioral variables, all having the field of action in the diencephalon. The psychiatric nurse clinician intervenes directly or indirectly to alleviate disabling symptoms central to depression. As identified by Akiskal and McKinney (1975) these target symptoms are: nonrelatedness, anhedonia, hopelessness, alterations in functional levels of biogenic amines, electrolyte disturbances, vegetative dysfunctions, and psychomotor dysfunctions.

Critical to this data collection and assessment step is identification of patient strengths that may impact later decision points. What is referred to by "patient strengths" is not, for example, the patient's ability to attend classes of some sort or complete an occupational therapy project. Patient strengths refer to personality strengths that make the aforementioned activities possible. Paolino (1981) outlined patient strengths relevant to verbal therapy; the author has elaborated on this list:

1. Capacity for psychological mindedness and insight, i.e., the ability to think about what one observes in self.
2. Capacity to tolerate anxiety, depression, and other painful feelings and thoughts.
3. Intelligence.
4. A relative mastery of early trauma or deprivation.
5. Capacity to develop trust and mutuality in interpersonal relationships.
6. Capacity for self-discipline.
7. Desire for less emotional pain.
8. Capacity to experience feelings rather than to just describe them.
9. Capacity for humor.
10. Capacity to be flexible.
11. Capacity for empathy towards others.
12. Capacity to engage others via effective communication.
13. Capacity for hope.

Any of the above strengths present in the individual can help facilitate treatment endeavors and should be capitalized upon whenever feasible.

STEP 2. OBTAIN THE PATIENT'S PLAN

The initial step in the process of differential therapeutics begins with obtaining the patient's treatment plan. The patient's ideas of what he or she wants to achieve in treatment, as well as how she or he feels these can be achieved, is the

---

*The reader is referred to other sources (Wilson, et. al, 1983 and Stuart et. al 1983) for nursing assessments of depression.

Table 8-1   Interventions for Provision of Safety: Management of the Psychiatric Crisis

Nonspecific psychiatric nursing practices	Psychiatric nursing practices specifically related to pharmacotherapy	Utilization of self-help activities/lay helping network
Monitor and/or intervene in medical crisis	Monitor and/or intervene in medical crisis involving drug overdose or drug toxicity.	Utilize family or other support systems in the service of protecting patient and/or others from injury.
Utilize verbal crisis intervention techniques with focus on the present.	Administer STAT medications as ordered.	
Maintain safe environment	Utilize efficient, nonpunitive therapeutic approaches to administering STAT medications.	
Prevent self-injury and injury to others.		
Communicate empathic acceptance of patients and their delusions and/or hallucinations.		
Assist patient in reality orientation.		
Mobilize additional professional assistance.		
Maintain low stimulus environment.		
Mobilize previous strengths and coping mechanisms.		
Allow patient to exercise as much control in situation as he or she is able to.		
Ensure availability of someone present with patient.		

recommended beginning point. Surely any treatment objective or plan of action not desired to some degree by the patient will ultimately result in failure. The nurse clinician may simply initiate the dialogue by asking "How do you feel we may be of help to you?" and "What do you hope to gain from treatment here?" Keeping in mind the patient's response, the nurse clinician now makes an independent analysis in the following Steps 3, 4, and 5.

Table 8-2   Interventions for Immediate Control of Disabling Symptoms

Non-specific psychiatric nursing practices	Psychiatric nursing practices specifically related to pharmacotherapy	Utilization of self-help activities/lay helping network
Establish and maintain adequate biological functioning in areas of sleep, nutrition and elimination.	Monitor effectiveness of pharmacotherapy.	Inform families of 24-hour emergency contact network.
Monitor for signs and symptoms of suicidal risk.	Recommend initiation of or changes in pharmacotherapy.	Provide guidance to family or appropriate others regarding management of patient at home.
Establish 24-hour emergency contact network.	Administer neuroleptics as ordered.	Utilize patient support systems as appropriate.
Monitor for presence of delusions and hallucinations.	Assess for acute side effects of medications.	
Alter external environment to prevent development of crisis.	Administer P.R.N. medications as ordered.	
Foster trusting nonjudgmental nurse-patient relationship.		
Give gentle reassurance that depressive symptomology will gradually abate.		
Establish and maintain adequate structured daily activity levels.		
Assist patient to identify and utilize appropriate alternative for control of destructive impulses.		
Provide assistance with daily living activities as necessary.		
Provide opportunities for reality testing.		

STEP 3.   PROVIDE FOR PATIENT SAFETY: MANAGE THE PSYCHIATRIC CRISIS

Provision of safety is always the highest priority and merits immediate intervention. Out-patient clinicians must, at all times, consider this potential treatment need and respond appropriately. The severely depressed patient may require crisis intervention as a result of suicidal ideation or attempts, threats of harm to others, or gross inability to care for self. Inappropriate levels of psychotropic medications may also necessitate emergency interventions. Table 8-1 outlines typical nursing interventions for provision of safety objectives.

Safety needs in the psychiatric crisis is a special part of the main body of the process of differential therapeutics. Safety needs are separated out because of their emergency orientation. Whenever such safety needs are evident, the nurse bypasses Steps 4 and 5, which ascertain less acute treatment needs and methods, and proceeds directly to identification of a treatment setting in Step 6.

Assuming there are no life-threatening treatment needs, further identification of general approaches to treatment proceeds.

Table 8-3   Interventions for Provision of Life Necessities

Nonspecific psychiatric nursing practices	Psychiatric nursing practices specifically related to pharmacotherapy	Utilization of self-help activities/Lay-helping network
Identify and/or contact professional referral resources, e.g., government social welfare agencies, legal consultation, other health care providers.	Monitor availability of prescribed medications.	Identify community resources available for provision of food, shelter, and clothing.
Identify source of patient payment for current psychiatric/medical treatment.	Assist patient in seeking funds for prescribed medications.	Support and reinforce self-care behaviors.
Discuss financial concerns with patient and family.		
Assist patient with management of resources.		
Identify and discuss priorities		

Table 8-4   Interventions for Provision of Information/ Patient Teaching

Nonspecific psychiatric nursing practices	Psychiatric nursing practices specifically related to pharmacotherapy	Utilization of self-help activities/lay helping network
Provide holistic explanation of depression Encourage patient questions. Provide information as appropriate regarding treatments for depression. For discharge planning, evaluate patient awareness of worsening or reoccurrence of symptoms.	Provide simple explanations regarding reasons for pharmacotherapy. Provide patient with realistic expectations of timeframe for medications to take effect. Provide information regarding side effects and their treatment. Identify problems in medication compliance. Evaluate patient comprehension of medication administration, e.g., dosages, dosage schedule, identification of pills, and side effects. Encourage self-responsibility in medication compliance. Refer patient to medication group.	Provide information to family or close supports as appropriate.

Table 8-5   Interventions for Support or Maintenance of Current or Past Levels of Adjustment

Nonspecific psychiatric nursing practices	Psychiatric nursing practices specifically related to pharmacotherapy	Formal psychotherapy	Utilization of self-help activities/lay helping network
Reduce excessive demands placed on patient.	Reinforce necessity for follow-up appointments.	Refer to or initiate Supportive Individual Psychotherapy or Supportive Group Therapy to achieve any of the following:	Support and reinforce self-care behaviors.
Encourage striving for realistic goals.	Monitor patient compliance with pharmacotherapy.		Encourage problem-solving with other patients.
Avoid direct challenge of patient defenses.	Monitor and intervene in side effects.	• decrease anxiety or fear	Encourage social activities.
Give positive encouragement for therapeutic gains.	Monitor current dosages and blood levels.	• strengthen existing defenses	Encourage family shared responsibilities.
Foster consistent and trusting nurse–patient relationship.	Encourage and respond to patient verbalizations of concerns regarding pharmacotherapy.	• promote better adaptation to the environment	Encourage utilization of community resources.
Encourage expression and working through of feelings.	Refer patient to medication group.	• maintain professional support network	
Develop alternative coping mechanisms.		• share situational difficulties as they arise with opportunity to problem solve	
Mobilize and redirect anger.		• provide and maintain satisfying relations with others	
Interrupt and reality test excessive rumination of negative thoughts.			

Nonspecific psychiatric nursing practices	Psychiatric nursing practices specifically related to pharmacotherapy	Formal psychotherapy	Utilization of self-help activities/lay helping network
Assist patient to structure daily activity.		• relief of a specific difficulty (e.g., deficit in social skills, need for increased assertiveness, etc.)	
Encourage physical activity.			
Encourage gradual resumption of previous productivity.		• validation of self-worth	
Increase patient awareness of behavior.			
Reality test feelings of guilt.			
Assist patient in developing problem solving skills.			
Refer patient for activity therapy groups such as poetry therapy, art therapy, music therapy, dance therapy.			
Refer patient for occupational or recreational therapy groups.			
Assist patient to identify and engage in pleasurable activities.			

STEP 4.   IDENTIFY GENERAL TREATMENT OBJECTIVES

The author has formulated nine treatment approaches available in out-patient settings:

Provision of safety: management of the psychiatric crisis (Refer to Step 3.).

Immediate control or relief of disabling symptoms (Table 8-2). Clusters of depressive symptoms may have severely debilitating effects for which specific interventions must be immediately targeted. Such symptoms, e.g., sleep disturbances with an inability to arise in the mornings and extreme lethargy, may impair access to needed treatment. Hopelessness and despair may portend suicidal ideation if relief is not soon forthcoming. Such situations merit this treatment approach.

Availability and/or provision of life necessities (Table 8-3). Life necessities include food, clothing, and shelter. There may be instances that certainly can never be overlooked, in which basic survival conditions are significantly contributory to the depression. Income maintenance, accessibility to health care and legal protection are also subsumed under this approach.

Provision of information/patient teaching (Table 8-4). Providing the patient and family with necessary information regarding assessment and treatment communicates the expectation that the patient is a full participant in treatment. Treatment is not shrouded in mystery nor under undisputed control by higher authority figures.

Support or maintenance of current or past levels of adjustment (Table 8-5). This treatment approach is an intermediate one between the acute and the more intensive treatment objectives designed for longer term effects. Restoration of pre-depression levels of adequate functioning represents short-term objectives. Krauss and Slavinsky (1982) state: "Sustaining current or past levels of adjustment requires strengthening existing ego defenses, stabilizing or restoring intrapsychic equilibrium as rapidly as possible and solidifying assets or recent therapeutic gains".

Individual personal reconstruction (Table 8-6). The term *reconstruction* will refer to interventions designed to facilitate self-understanding and self-awareness that find expression through changes in values and attitudes, through personality and behavioral changes, and development of more effective coping styles. Psychotherapy has its main focus in this area.

Development of improved interpersonal behavior patterns (Table 8-7). The goal of improving interpersonal relationships encompasses a wide spectrum of interventions, e.g., alleviating depression via enhancing family

Table 8-6   Interventions for Individual Personal Reconstruction

Nonspecific psychiatric nursing practices	Formal psychotherapy	Utilization of self-help activities/lay helping networks
Recognize loss and its meaning to patient.	Initiate individual psychotherapy to achieve any of the following:	Support and reinforce self-care behaviors.
Encourage expression and working through of feelings.	• relief of a specific symptom	Encourage patient to test new perceptions, responses with family, friends, work acquaintances, etc.
Identify self-esteem needs.	• correct erroneous perceptions by reconstructing or reenacting the past	Encourage utilization of self-help groups as appropriate (e.g., Al-anon), lay support groups for particular problems (e.g., single parent groups).
Encourage awareness of self-deception.		
Assist patient to identify problematic emotional patterns.	• change behavior through strengthening control	
Explore personality strengths and weaknesses.	• become aware of and practice new patterns of interpersonal behavior	
Challenge defenses.	• catharsis to relieve intensity of emotions	
Reinforce ownership of consequences of own behavior.	• decrease irrational beliefs through cognitive retraining	
Foster independence of thought and action.	• reintegrate mind and body (feelings and viscera)	
Provide opportunities for and encourage responsible roles.	• increase satisfaction in interpersonal relationships	
Assist patient to develop congruence between verbal and nonverbal systems.	• decrease individual excessive denial of responsibility for own behavior which has stalemated family therapy or group therapy	
Refer to activity therapy groups such as poetry therapy, art therapy, music therapy, dance therapy		

Table 8-7   Interventions for Improved Interpersonal Behavior Patterns

Nonspecific psychiatric nursing practices	Formal psychotherapy	Utilization of self-help activities/lay helping networks
Foster trusting nurse–patient relationship.	Refer to or initiate <u>group therapy</u> to achieve any of the following:	Encourage practice of new interpersonal skills with family, friends, etc.
Provide opportunities for corrective social interactions.	• increase satisfaction in interpersonal interactions	Encourage utilization of self-help groups as appropriate.
Assist patient to identify problematic areas in interpersonal functioning.	• receive feedback regarding dysfunctional interpersonal skills	Encourage outside social activities such as church groups, volunteer work, or dating.
Encourage verbal participation in groups.	• have opportunity to share one's self to help another	Encourage family shared responsibilities.
Encourage active participation in therapeutic milieu.	• increase assertiveness	
Encourage increased risk taking in interpersonal interactions.	• experience sense of community or belonging	
Role model or role play appropriate social interactions.	• decrease anxiety or shyness in interpersonal interactions	
Encourage assertiveness.	• increase mutuality in relationships via greater awareness of own and other's feelings	
Facilitate clear family communications.	• exposure to role models	
Encourage suitable levels of independence/dependence upon family.	Refer to or initiate <u>family therapy</u> or marital therapy to achieve any of the following:	
	• opening communication within the family	
	• build self-esteem within the family	
	• develop more satisfying and/or supporting	

Nonspecific psychiatric nursing practices	Formal psychotherapy	Utilization of self-help activities/lay helping networks
	roles or family relations	
	• learn and practice clearer communication among family unit	
	• foster individuality within the family unit	
	• improvement of patient via other forms of treatment has led to deterioration in other family members	
	• address patients' primary concerns of family issues which cannot be met via other forms of treatment	

interactions, or facilitating improved communication and social skills in a group therapy context.

Rehabilitation (Table 8-8).   Bozarth et al. (1976) describe the overall treatment goal of psychiatric rehabilitation as a gradual training process, helping the patient to ". . . perform the physical, intellectual, and emotional skills needed to live, learn, and work in his or her particular community, given the least amount of support necessary from agents of the helping professions." This process may occur outside the confines of a psychiatric mental health facility and as part of community involvment, such as YMCA/YWCA programs, sheltered workshops, vocational testing and training, and volunteer placements. Residential facilities such as group homes, board and care, or half-way houses also apply to psychiatric rehabilitation. The chronic depressive patients in the community have been largely unrecognized and hence poorly treated (Weissman & Klerman, 1977 and Weisman & Kasl, 1976). This particular group of patients may require this type of treatment approach.

Broadening the scope of participation in life (Table 8-9).   This category of intervention approaches is aimed at expanding and improving the quality of the individual's pre-depression life-style. This may include such interventions as encouraging participation in sports, taking music lessons, joining new clubs,

Table 8-8   Interventions for Rehabilitation*

Nonspecific psychiatric nursing practices	Psychiatric nursing practices specifically related to pharmacotherapy	Formal psychotherapy	Utilization of self-help activities/lay helping network
Encourage gradual mastery of social or physical difficulties. Encourage striving for realistic goals. Facilitate recognition and acceptance of a chronic illness. Assist patient in meeting essential living needs. Identify professional resources for crisis support. Offer advice and guidance. Refer patient to occupational or recreational therapy groups. Refer patient to pre-vocational or vocational training. Assist patient in identifying and engage in pleasurable activities. Assist patient in identifying signs and symptoms of reoccuring depression.	Give verbal reassurance. Monitor maintenance therapy of antidepressants. Monitor for potential ineffective pharmacotherapy of minor tranquilizers and maintenance antipsychotics. Monitor for side effects. Reinforce necessity for medication follow-up appointments.	Refer to or initiate supportive individual psychotherapy or supportive group therapy to achieve any of the following: • decrease fear or anxiety • on-going assessment for reoccurence of depressive symptomology • tolerate unalterable situations • promote better adaptation to environment • provide positive encouragement from others • provide opportunity for on-going reality testing	Support and reinforce self-care behaviors. Identify and/or contact community resources as necessary, e.g. volunteer work or placements. Encourage development of supportive peer relationships. Refer patient to supportive/structured living environment as needed.

*See also Table 8-7.

Table 8-9   Interventions for Broadening the Scope of Participation in Life

Nonspecific psychiatric nursing practices	Formal psychotherapy	Utilization of self-help activities/lay helping networks
Encourage evaluation of therapeutic goals.	Begin and complete termination phase of individual or group psychotherapy.	Encourage risk taking in interpersonal relationships.
Emphasize independence of thought and action.	Recommend "no treatment" as treatment of choice.	Encourage development of new interests.
Encourage decreasing reliance on professional help (facilitate process of patient becoming "own therapist").		Encourage utilization of community resources such as school, employment, etc.
Communicate confidence in patient's personal strengths and resources.		Encourage development of a reliable, supportive, helping network.
Encourage exploration of long-range life goals.		Recommend self-help aides such as books, e.g., *Feeling Good* (Burns, 1980).
Recommend "no treatment" as treatment of choice.		

developing hobbies, pursing intellectual endeavors, and generally investing energy in heretofore unknown or inexperienced areas of life. Depressions involving significant losses often create major alterations in an individual's former way of life, necessitating examination of alternatives to living.

These treatment approaches are not mutually exclusive. Furthermore, any one of them may encompass interventions for experiential, chemical, and behavioral aspects of depression. This identification of general approaches begins the process of defining, refining, and selecting an appropriate treatment plan.

STEP 5.   CHOOSE THE TREATMENT MODALITY: DIFFERENTIAL THERAPEUTICS

Step 5 is the core of differential therapeutics. It is here that the nurse clinician must visualize all treatment alternatives and decide how most effectively to intervene to meet the identified objectives chosen in Step 4.

All therapeutic modalities utilized by psychiatric nurse clinicians are encompassed in one or more of the following categories:

Nonspecific psychiatric nursing practices.   This category includes general psychiatric nursing care that can be found in any current, comprehensive textbook on psychiatric nursing. The practice applies to all levels of academically prepared nurses. Indeed, nurses with specialist degrees or training (e.g., a nurse psychotherapist) will invariably utilize many of the strategies from this category.

Psychiatric nursing practices specifically related to pharmacotherapy.   This category is a subset of the previous one but it is discussed separately to accentuate its importance. Nurses' training differs from that of many other mental health professionals' in its additional focus upon the chemical aspects of depression. This training allows the nurse clinician to more accurately monitor drug effectiveness, to make recommendations that could initiate, enhance, or terminate drug therapy, to administer medications, to intervene in the development of side effects, and to provide patient teaching regarding medications. Any one of these nursing interventions will serve to increase patient compliance with pharmacotherapy. Pharmacotherapy, along with the psychotherapies, represents the major class of treatment modalities most often researched in comparative efficacy studies.

Formal psychotherapy.   The psychiatric nurse may refer a patient for such services or may have advanced degrees or training to deliver these specialized services personally. All available forms of psychotherapy may be classified under individual, group, or family therapy. These may be further classified into particular ''brands'' or schools or psychotherapy.

Self-help activities/Lay helping networks.   This diverse category will encompass: (1) employment as a therapeutic force; (2) participation in community and social activities such as volunteer work or involvement in community organizations; (3) utilization of self-help groups; (4) reliance on family and friends networks; and (5) positive, unidentified therapeutic movements that occur in the context of either no treatment from professional clinicians or so-called ''spontaneous improvement'' that may occur in control groups of experimental studies as the result of the placebo effect.

For each general treatment objective identified in Step 4, the nurse clinician now chooses appropriate interventions from among the four nurse practice treatment modalities (See Table 8-10). Careful consideration of interventions in each of the relevant treatment modality categories will yield the most comprehensive treatment plan.

Suggested nursing interventions for each general treatment objective are listed in Tables 8-1 through 8-9. This list is not exhaustive but attempts to incorporate the most typically utilized treatments for depression across all outpatient settings. Some of the interventions, of course, may be more applicable in one setting than another.

Table 8-10   Psychiatric Nursing Treatment Modalities

Treatment objectives	Treatment modalities			
	Nonspecific psychiatric nursing practices	Psychiatric nursing practices specifically related to pharmaco-therapy	Formal psycho-therapy	Utilization of self-help activities/lay helping network
Provision of safety				
1. Management of psychiatric crisis	X	X		X
2. Immediate control of disabling symptoms	X	X		X
3. Availability and/or provision of life necessities	X	X		X
4. Provision of information: patient teaching	X	X		X
5. Support of maintenance of current or past levels of adjustment	X	X	X	X
6. Rehabilitation	X	X	X	X
7. Individual personal reconstruction	X		X	X
8. Development of improved interpersonal behavior patterns	X		X	X
9. Broadening the scope of participation in life	X		X	X

143

Treatment Decisions Based Upon Research

Nursing is an applied science that relies on the continued generation and/or awareness of new knowledge derived from clinical investigation, either in nursing or from other disciplines. Nurses base clinical practice not only upon recent research outcomes but also upon their past clinical experiences of trial and error. In areas not validated by these two methods nurses must depend upon intuition and common sense. The latter two components of decision-making mechanisms (i.e., reliance upon past experiences and common sense) are by no means negligible aspects, particularly in the field of psychiatry where such a large number of variables impinge on a clinical decision.

The effectiveness of nonspecific psychiatric nursing practices has been validated primarily through clinical practice. In the research literature, formal psychotherapies and pharmacotherapy have received the most attention in research comparisons. What has been delineated as the self-help activities/lay-helping network category has received some commentary, largely from studies comparing psychotherapy groups to no psychotherapy groups (i.e., control groups).

No Professional Treatment

All research evidence suggests a rather clear-cut case for the efficacy of psychotherapy or pharmacotherapy as opposed to the absence of these treatments. Despite the fact that spontaneous remissions are less frequent than once purported to be, nurse clinicians cannot ignore this phenomenon. Some degree of "spontaneous improvement" does, in fact, occur in patients who do not receive formal treatment. This undefined positive effect may be the result of potent therapeutic sources outside professional auspices. Indeed, helping networks available to patients include both the "professional" and "natural" networks (Naparstek, 1977). The professional network includes mental health centers, general hospitals, public welfare agencies, courts, schools, religious institutions, nursing homes, emergency/crisis services, private practice services, social service agencies, and child guidance centers. The "natural" or lay-helping networks include family, friends, neighbors, self-help groups, teachers, voluntary organizations, and other informal helpers. Although within the context of a professional network, fellow patients, in milieu settings, group therapies, etc., must also be considered a powerful therapeutic lay-network force.

The recognition and subsequent utilization of self-help activities and the lay helping networks will be a significant adjunct to professional treatment.

The decision for no treatment by professional intervention has been thoughtfully reviewed by Frances and Clarkin (1981b). They discuss research methodology and problems inherent in defining those patients who are better off without treatment. Their review of literature generates the following patient groups in which treatment is either harmful or unnecessary:

1. Negative responders
    *   patients prone to severe negative therapeutic reactions such as masochistic, narcissistic and/or oppositional personality disorders.
    *   patients who enter treatment primarily to justify a claim for compensation or disability, or to support a lawsuit.
2. Nonresponders
    *   chronically dependent, treatment-addicted patients.
    *   patients with antisocial or criminal behavior.
    *   patients with factitious illness.
    *   patients who are poorly motivated and without incapacitating symptoms.
3. Spontaneous Improvers
    *   patients in the midst of a grief reaction or crisis who have sufficient psychological and social network resources available to them.
    *   patients who are generally healthy.

In any of the aforementioned groups, the choice for no treatment may serve to:

. . . (1) protect the patient from iatrogenic harm (particularly to interrupt a sequence of destructive treatments); (2) protect the patient (and clinician) from wasting time, effort, and money; (3) delay therapy until a more propitious time; (4) protect and consolidate gains from a previous treatment; (5) provide the patient an opportunity to discover that he can do without treatment; and (6) avoid a semblance of treatment when no effective treatment exists.

Nurse clinicians, whether they be directly or indirectly involved in the decision for no treatment, need to acknowledge this as a viable treatment decision.

In summary, two points must not be overlooked in our current practices: (1) Absence of professional treatment does not preclude therapeutic activity; and (2) Within the context of professional treatment, utilization of non-professional therapeutic activities or networks is likely to enhance treatment outcome.

Pharmacotherapy and Psychotherapy

Continuing on in the selection of treatment modalities based upon research, the nurse clinician may query how effective pharmacotherapy is versus psychotherapy in the treatment of depressed out-patients. Whether individual, or group, or family therapy is most effective, and which "brand" or school of psychotherapy works best.

The most extensive surveys of comparative efficacy studies of psychotherapy and pharmacotherapy appear in three major works; the Luborsky et al. study (1975), Garfield and Bergin, (1978), and Smith et al. (1980). Unfortunately, in these collective surveys, little effort was made to delineate research studies that applied to any one diagnostic category. In fact, many of the surveyed

Table 8-11 Research on Cognitive Therapy and Behavior Therapy

Investigators and References	Groups treatment	Sample	Outcome
Rush et al. (1977)	Cognitive therapy vs. imipramine	Unipolar N=41	Cognitive therapy showed more improvement and less attrition than imipramine
Shaw (1977)	Cognitive therapy vs. behavior therapy vs. assessment attention vs. waiting list	Depressed N=32	Cognitive therapy resulted in the most effectiveness in alleviating depression. All groups resulted in fewer symptoms than waiting list. No differences found between behavior therapy and nondirective assessment/attention group
Taylor (1977)	Cognitive and behavioral vs. cognitive vs. behavioral vs. waiting list	Depressed N=28	No significant differences between behavioral and cognitive treatments. Combination more effective than either alone; all treatments better than waiting list.
Zeiss et al. (1979)	Interpersonal behavior modality vs. pleasant events schedule modality vs. cognitive modality	Depressed N=66	No significant differences between cognitive and behavioral treatments. All treatments were effective in alleviating depression. No treatment modality had specific impact on variables most relevant to its treatment format.

Study	Treatment comparison	Population	Results
McLean and Hakstian (1979)	Psychotherapy vs. behavior therapy vs. drug therapy vs. relaxation therapy (control)	Depressed N=178	Behavior therapy resulted in less attrition and more improvement over all treatment groups. Psychotherapy performed most poorly; no significant difference between drug therapy and relaxation therapy.
Wilson et al. (1983)	Behavior vs. cognitive vs. no treatment of depression	Depressed N=25	Cognitive and behavioral treatment showed equal effectiveness in alleviating depression. Either were more effective than no treatment.
Bellak et al. (1983)	Amitriptyline vs. social skills training (SST) plus amitriptyline vs. SST plus placebo vs. psychotherapy plus placebo	Depressed unipolar N=125	All groups produced significant changes in symptomology. SST groups had greater improvement on measures of social skill, SST plus placebo group had lowest attrition with highest proportion of patients who improved.
Rehm et al. (1979)	Assertion skills group vs. self-control condition	Depressed N=124	Self-control groups improved more on measures of self-control, assertion skills; group improved more on assertion skills measures; self-control groups improved more in alleviating depression.

Adapted from Weissman, M. (1979) The psychological treatment of depression. *Archives of General Psychiatry, 36*, 1261–1269. Copyright 1979, American Medical Association. With permission.

experimental studies themselves did not seek to test a homogeneous sample of subjects. It is interesting to note, however, that many of the results (Epstein, et. al. 1981; Smith, 1982) generally are in concurrence with conclusions based upon the studies that appear in Tables 8-11, 8-12, and 8-13 that tested only depressed populations. Although no reviews of the three studies will be given here, the reader is referred to them for further valuable comparisons of treatment outcome.

In attempting to limit research studies that have clinical experimental trials of out-patient depressed subjects (omitting single-case studies and comparative treatment studies without random assignment in controlled clinical trials), the pool of research becomes quite small. Only five psychotherapy treatment modalities have been subject to comparative experimental trials. These are psychotherapy, cognitive, behavioral, group, and marital therapy.

The psychotherapy category actually encompasses more than 140 different approaches or "brands." Weissman (1979) has globally defined psychotherapy as:

. . . a confiding relationship and a verbal dialogue between the person administering the treatment and the person receiving it. This dialogue is specifically directed at bringing about a desired psychological and/or social change in the recipient; e.g., reduction of symptoms, improved adaptation, better social functioning, increased self-esteem, and more assertiveness.

Cognitive therapy is, of course, a form of psychotherapy, but is a treatment generally administered on a short-term basis in which principally didactic explanations and cognitive tasks are given to correct the depressed patient's negative thinking and attitudes (Beck et al., 1979 and Rush, et. al, 1981).

Behavior therapy, based upon the principles of stimulus/response theory, utilizes positive reinforcers to shape desired behaviors. Several techniques based on behavioral concepts that have been identified have been employed in the treatment of depression (Bellack, et. al. 1979; Hersen, et. al. 1978; Weissman, 1979; Williams, 1984). Among them are:

. . . 1) Social skills therapy, which emphasizes increasing assertiveness, verbal skills, and social adjustments, 2) activity scheduling of pleasant events, which focus on increasing pleasant and rewarding experiences; and 3) contingency management which emphasizes self-monitoring, self-control, self-evaluation and reinforcement to interrupt the exclusive focus upon negative events and excessive self-punishment.

Tables 8-11 through 8-13 summarize the results from current research, testing treatment modality efficacy for out-patient depressed clients.

Based upon limited current research, several general statements may be made regarding the efficacy of treatment modalities for depressed patients:

1.   Psychotherapy and pharmacotherapy are effective treatments for depression and each is superior to no treatment.

2.   There is some evidence for the beneficial combination of psychotherapy and pharmacotherapy.

Table 8-12   Research on Drug Therapy and Psychotherapy

Investigators and References	Groups treatment	Sample	Outcome
Klerman et al. (1974)	Drugs vs. psychotherapy vs. drugs and psychotherapy	Depressed females N=150	No differences between drug therapy alone or drug therapy with psychotherapy. Drug reduced relapse rate.
Weissman et al. (1979) Rounsaville et al. (1980)	Psychotherapy alone vs. pharmacotherapy vs. psychotherapy plus pharmacotherapy vs. nonscheduled treatment	Depressed unipolar N=97	Pharmacotherapy and psychotherapy alone were equally effective; each was better than nonscheduled treatment. Combination of psychotherapy and pharmacotherapy was more effective than either treatment alone.

Adapted from Weissman, M. (1979) The psychological treatment of depression. *Archives of General Psychiatry, 36,* 1261–1269. Copyright 1979, American Medical Association. With permission.

Table 8-13   Research on Group Therapy and Conjoint Marital Therapy

Investigators and References	Groups treatment	Sample	Outcome
Covi et al. (1974)	Drug (imipramine vs. diazepam vs. placebo) plus group psychotherapy or brief supportive psychiatric contact	Depressed chronic females N=146	Imipramine was superior to other drug treatments. No advantage for group therapy over brief supportive psychiatric contact. Weak effect occurred late for group therapy.
Sanchez et al. (1980)	Group assertion training vs. traditional group psychotherapy	Depressed N=32	Group assertion training was more effective than traditional group psychotherapy in increasing assertiveness and in alleviating depression.
Friedman (1975)	Drug-marital therapy vs. drug-minimal contact vs. placebo-martial therapy vs. placebo minimal contact.	Depressed married N=196	Drug and martial therapy each showed effectiveness over controls. Drug therapy had early effect to reduce hostility and enhance perception of marital relationship; Marital therapy had a late effect but superior effect on family role task performance and perception of martial relationship.

Adapted from Weissman, M. (1979) The psychological treatment of depression. *Archives of General Psychiatry, 36*, 1261–1269. Copyright 1979, American Medical Association. With permission.

3.   Psychotherapy as compared to pharmacotherapy may produce more improved social functioning effects.

4.   There is some indication that the therapeutic effects of group and marital therapy occur later in treatment.

5.   Cognitive therapy and behavioral therapies, without pharmacotherapy or in combination with pharmocotherapy, are effective modalities in the treatment of depression (Kovacs, 1980).

6.   A large number of schools of psychotherapy have yet to be subjected to rigorous comparative efficacy studies with depressed patient populations.

The nurse clinician utilizes this knowledge to give partial validation to her or his practice. These are not meant to be prescriptions for treatment, but areas for impact upon the decision-making process. Traditional wisdom still must be relied upon for selecting specific treatment modalities for targeted treatment objectives (Clarkin, 1979; Frances, et. al., 1980; Grunebaum, et. al., 1977). Characteristic withdrawal from and difficulties with interpersonal relationships, e.g., self defeatism and chronic submissiveness, may be effectively treated in group therapy; disrupted family relations that either preceded or were the consequence of depression may indicate the need for family therapy. However, research findings may guide nursing practices to specialized areas of treatment, e.g., even though a nurse clinician may not be well-versed in administering formal behavioral therapy or cognitive therapy, he or she may apply various components of these therapies in practice, including cognitive approaches to invalidate persistent negative thoughts or role-playing effective assertive skills or assisting the patient to identify and engage in pleasurable activities.

Several reasons that caution must be exercised against wholesale transfer of these research implications onto clinical practice are (1) the comparative research studies are few in number and require more duplication to increase validity; (2) only a few therapeutic modalities out of more than a hundred varieties have been researched; (3) there is an increasing blending of therapeutic schools of psychotherapy, both theoretically in the newer schools as well as in eclectic approaches to practice by clinicians; and (4) patients often have multiple diagnoses and personality make-up that may render the recommended treatments either inapplicable or short-sighted.

After the nurse clinician has decided upon the preferred treatment modalities for each treatment objective, he or she combines these with the patient's own stated objectives and desired methods.

STEP 6:   IDENTIFY THE TREATMENT SETTING

Loosely construed as being any treatment setting not of an in-patient hospital nature, out-patient treatment settings are quite varied. There are partial hospitalization programs, the lay-community or "natural" therapeutic settings, psychiatric out-patient departments of hospitals, community mental health centers, private practice facilities not associated with hospitals, residential facilities (e.g., psychiatric boarding homes, and group homes), and school counseling centers. In-patient hospitalization may be included as a necessary sequel to out-patient treatment under conditions where 24-hour surveillance is required.

Generalizations concerning differences between treatment settings are difficult to make. Individual programs within a setting category may differ significantly from each other or there may be extensive category overlap. Each program must be evaluated separately on the basis of (1) type and scope of services offered; (2) type of patients accepted; (3) usual duration of treatment; (4) program hours; (5) qualification of clinicians; (6) fees; (7) quality of the services offered; (8) availability of emergency services; and (9) location of facility for patient accessibility. Any sweeping differentiation of treatment settings based upon scope, quality or types of services would be difficult if not wholly inaccurate. It would be at least acceptable to most clinicians to outline a setting continuum based upon the level of patient functioning appropriate to each setting. The level of patient functioning determines the amount of programmatic structure required and amount of responsibility for treatment a patient must assume. Table 8-14 offers a list of treatment settings appropriate for patients with lowest to highest levels of functioning.

The continuum in Table 8-14 has implications for time sequencing dependent upon changes in patient levels of functioning. In predicting and evaluating treatment outcomes, the clinician must anticipate possible movements from one setting to another. One patient may move from a community mental health facility to a partial hospitalization program during worsening of illness, but return to the community mental health center after the crisis has been averted. Another patient may be hospitalized and then referred to an out-patient department while he or she resumes prior employment with eventual reliance upon nonprofessional community supports.

There may be times when multiple-setting use is indicated. One patient may reside in a residential facility but spend his days at a partial hospital program. Another patient may have only a monthly follow-up to the out-patient clinic; her "treatment" largely occurs in the lay community.

The nurse clinician must ask the patient for any feelings he or she may have

Table 8-14   Psychiatric Treatment Settings

Patient functioning	Highest --- Lowest							
Treatment setting	Lay Community	School counseling center	Private practice facility	Community mental health center	Psychiatric out-patient clinic of hospital	Residential facility	Partial hospital program	In-patient unit

regarding a particular treatment setting. Prior experience with an agency or program may steer the decision for treatment away or towards it.

At this point, the nurse and patient will review the assessment, preferred treatment modalities, and recommended treatment setting.

STEP 7. NEGOTIATE

Orlinsky and Howard (1978) portray rather incisively the most commonly practiced process by which treatment plans are generated:

> Generally the normative organization of therapeutic process is unilaterally deter-
> mined by the therapist's precription, with the patient's negotiative options reduced to
> acceptance or refusal of the therapist's terms (when treatment is voluntary).
>
> If the therapist allows it, there may be some negotiation over fees, hours, and
> frequency of visits. If the patient wills it, a covert resistance against the arrangement can
> be maintained. The therapist's authority as a socially sanctioned specialist is further
> reinforced by the power imbalance that is created by the patient's state of need and the
> relative supply and demand for therapeutic services.

Nursing, based in the principles of symbolic interaction, seeks greater negotiation between therapist and patient. As Orlinsky and Howard (1978) imply, passive compliance or outright resistance are risks one imposes upon treatment via the normative organization approach. Nurse clinicians need to be cognizant of patient "prescriptions" and preferences during formulation of the plans. Out of this will arise dialogues between two active participants as they listen, exchange ideas, modify, receive feedback, compromise or renegotiate—all of which are of themselves therapeutic processes.

Whenever possible, unless safety issues preclude a patient's participation in treatment planning, the nurse clinician must support the patients' self-direction. For every treatment decision, there is an alternative and hence an area for negotiation. There may be negotiations as to which facility to use, how many days a week, for how long, and for which days, and which groups. The patient may opt to "try out" a program before committing to a decision. For every level of motivation, there is a treatment plan that can be designed, however limited and within the bounds of safe, clinical practice. If the patient refuses all alternatives then this also must be respected.

In such negotiations, it is important that two conditions be upheld: the plans are mutually acceptable to both patient and clinician, and the patient and clinician are accountable to the terms agreed upon.

This process of negotiation in the generation of a treatment plan respects the patient as an individual with choice and responsibility for determining the direction of treatment and allows the nurse clinician to be a role model of flexibility and creativity.

STEP 8.   CLINICAL UNCERTAINTIES

The next series of steps are additional factors to treatment planning which, if not considered by the clinician, may jeopardize an otherwise well-constructed treatment plan.

Perceived Risks and Barriers

Barriers, risks, and costs are based upon personal value systems so that estimates of treatment costs may differ between patient and nurse clinician. Perceived personal barriers or costs may include such factors as the lack of guarantee of therapy outcome, time involved before antidepressant medications reach therapeutic thresholds, experiencing of psychological pain (such as fear or anxiety) during treatment, potential side effects of medications, and perhaps incurring the social stigma of psychiatric treatment. Pragmatic difficulties that may present as barriers may encompass seemingly trivial costs, such as commuting time to the treatment facility or arrangments for child care. Another significant consideration may be lack of support from family.

The financial cost of treatment is almost always a serious consideration of the patient. Transportation expenses, time off from work for treatment, baby-sitting fees, and all treatment expenses incurred beyond what is covered by health insurance (and these are often enormous), are all extra expenditures in the daily life of the patient. The patient and the nurse clinician may need to scrutinize this carefully when planning a feasible treatment. The nurse clinician in her practical orientation should not fail to address these seemingly trivial or "extra therapeutic" considerations. To construe them as part and parcel of "resistances" or some therapeutic issue is to repudiate them as real and integral aspects of a patient's daily life. Patients need to maintain financial stability in their strivings for health. The nurse clinician may direct the patient to special funding sources, assist in problem-solving on budget matters, or present alternatives to the treatment plan.

Particularly in the present national economic conditions, psychiatric nurses in all settings have become more involved in treatment funding matters. Demonstrating knowledge of specific insurance coverages, negotiating payment schedules, assisting patients in locating the most financially advantageous treatments, and assuming payment-collection responsibilities, may all be part of this expanded role.

Patient Motivation

As Frances and Clarkin (1981b) so aptly note "Motivation for treatment is always ambivalent; the most motivated have resistances, the least motivated may covertly beg for help."

Low patient motivation does not necessarily imply low treatability or vice versa. The match between the degree of patient motivation and the type of treatment offered is a critical consideration. Furthermore, motivation can change over time. For example, a patient is reluctant to engage in treatment but is offered a ''trial'' period during which time the patient's motivation increases as a result of the limited exposure to the treatment program. Another patient refuses group therapy, but will consider psychotherapy. Balancing the patient's motivation level with a suitable plan that adequately addresses the patient's needs requires both flexibility and creativity on the part of the nurse clinician.

For some patients who are poorly motivated and seem unwilling to invest in making changes in their lives, no treatment may indeed be the treatment of choice. A guide to this issue of no treatment is presented by Frances and Clarkin (1981b):

> In general, . . . treatment should not be sold or imposed on people who do not want it, except under the following conditions: (1) treatment is necessary to avoid considerable short- or long-term disability; (2) an effective treatment does not exist; and (3) because of his disorder, the patient is unable to make the most prudent decision without help.

Patient–Therapist Match

The nature of the patient–therapist match will exert a strong modifying effect upon motivation. Becker (1974) delineates the following factors that serve to create the initial impetus for treatment action on the part of the patient: (1) positive attitudes towards the visit in general, and towards the staff, clinic procedures, and facilities; (2) the quality of interaction with the helping professional; and (3) the type of patient–clinician relationship (clinician agreement with and feedback to the patient). In the vernacular of psychotherapy, the therapeutic alliance encapsulates these same factors. The perceived ''clinician agreement with the patient'' is likely to be an accurate acknowledgment of the patient's feelings. Patient drop-outs in treatment often can be attributed to the patient's ''not liking the therapist.'' Empathic listening and responding can serve the nurse clinician well to promote the needed motivation for treatment.

At times, the clinician may need to decide, for the welfare of that particular patient, to transfer or refer him or her to another clinician. Although rare, some patient problems may not be adequately treatable by a clinician due to personal reasons (e.g., counter-transference problems) or more likely because of the clinician not having a particular expertise in the treatment modality deemed most appropriate.

STEP 9. REVISE PLAN

Any revisions in the treatment plan based upon evaluation of clinical uncertainties are made at this point through a collaborative effort of the nurse, the patient, and the health-care team. As in Step 7, revision of the proposed treatment plan is also a therapeutic process.

The plan should now be reviewed and offered to the patient. If the patient does not agree to the plan, the nurse must back-track and attempt to ascertain whether any important aspects of the patient's self-assessment and preferred treatment plan were omitted. These must be integrated with the nurse's treatment plan. The nurse clinician will again make revisions in treatment setting or other aspects of the treatment plan based upon any newly discovered clinical uncertainties. It should be noted that one's initial assessment is not altered because the patient does not agree to the treatment contract.

If agreement to the plan is reached, continue to Step 10.

STEP 10. ARRANGE EVALUATION SCHEDULE

Research literature at this point in time gives the clinician little guidance in determining the most advantageous frequency and duration of psychotherapies and other treatments. Orlinsky and Howard (1978) sum up their results: ". . . More of a good thing is better than less of it; more of a bad thing is worse; and there may well be a point of diminishing returns . . . ."

In light of this nondefinitive prescription, the author recommends always establishing a specific time-frame to evaluate progress, be it in psychotherapy or a day-treatment program or family therapy. In addition, the nurse clinician will need to consider the patients' financial capabilities to sustain long-term treatments. The nurse must also assess the patients' potential for becoming overly dependent upon professional help at the expense of utilizing self and lay networks. Over-dependence upon professional assistance can evolve quite subtly in treatment. The nurse clinician can mitigate this tendency by actively supporting patient self-direction and self-responsibility from the start of treatment as well as by setting the mutually agreeable time frames for reassessment of goal attainment.

STEP 11. IMPLEMENT TREATMENT PLAN

The process of differential therapeutics has been completed at this step. Now follows implementation of the plan. At designated evaluation points in treatment or at points where treatment needs change dramatically, the whole process of differential therapeutics will again be initiated. At some points in treatment, this process will require little time; at other points, several meetings with the patient, health care professionals, and others will be necessitated.

SUMMARY

Differential therapeutics is a process that encompasses the assessment and planning portions of the nursing process. It is a process involving active participation of the patient, demands expert assessment skills, and knowledge of a variety of treatment modalities—with consideration of the practical concerns of daily living. Inherent in the out-patient treatment selection is the need to consistently reinforce the patient's self-direction and self-responsibility, and to utilize nonprofessional networks whenever feasible.

The process of differential therapeutics involves the following steps:

1. Assess for depression and other patient needs.
2. Obtain the patient's own ideas about treatment objectives and preferred methods of treatment.
3. Provide safety in the psychiatric crisis.
4. Identify general treatment goals.
5. Choose treatment modalities from among the four nurse-practice categories: nonspecific psychiatric nursing practices, psychiatric nursing practices specifically related to pharmacotherapy, formal psychotherapy, and self-help activities utilizing the lay helping networks.
6. Choose a treatment setting.
7. Offer a plan and negotiate.
8. Identify clinical uncertainties (i.e., perceived barriers to treatment).
9. Revise the plan as needed and offer the plan to patient.
10. Arrange an evaluation schedule.
11. Implement the plan of action.

The process of differential therapeutics described in this chapter, represents the comprehensive process by which experienced clinicians arrive at treatment plans. It is the systematic documentation of the "thinking process," as well as the collaborative steps involving the patient, by which the treatment plan is generated.

Clinical wisdom is often derived from repeated experience by doing. The neophyte is usually left to practice by imitation or to make clinical decisions based upon limited resources. This guide to the process of differential therapeutics has attempted to systematically document this process more accurately than "a pinch of this and a dash of that."

REFERENCES

Akiskal, H. S., & McKinney, W. T. (1975). Overview of recent research in depression. *Archives of General Psychiatry, 32,* 285–301.

Beck, A., Rush, A. J., Shaw, B. F., & Emery, G. (1979). *Cognitive therapy of depression.* New York: The Guilford Press.

Becker, M. H. (Ed.). (1974). *The health belief model and personal health behavior.* New Jersey: Charles B. Clack, Inc.

Bellack, A. S., & Hersen, M. (Eds.). (1979). *Research and practice in social skills training.* New York: Plenum Press.

Bellak, A. S., Hersen, M., & Himmelhock, J. M. (1983). A comparison of social-skills training, pharmacotherapy and psychotherapy for depression. *Behavior Research and Therapy, 21,*(2), 101–107.

Bozarth, J. D., & Rubin, S. E. (1976). Empirical observations of antecedants to psychotherapeutic outcome: Some implications. *Rehabilitation and Counseling Bulletin, 20,* (28), p. 30.

Burns, David D. (1980). *Feeling Good.* New York: The New American Library, Inc.

Clarkin, J. F., Frances, A. J., & Moodie, J. L. (1979). Selection criteria for family therapy. *Family Process, 18,* 391–403.

Covi, L., Lipman, R. S., Derogatis, L. R., Smith, J. E. III, & Pattison, J. H. (1974). Drugs and group psychotherapy in neurotic depression. *American Journal of Psychiatry, 131* (2), 191–198.

Epstein, N. B., & Vlok, L. A. (1981). Research on the results of psychotherapy: A summary of evidence. *American Journal of Psychiatry, 138* (8), 1027–1035.

Frances, A., & Clarkin, J. (1981a). Differential therapeutics: A guide to treatment selection. *Hospital and Community Psychiatry, 32* (8), 537–546.

Frances, A., & Clarkin, J. F. (1981b). No treatment as the prescription of choice. *Archives of General Psychiatry, 38,* 542–545.

Frances, A. F., & Marachi, J. P. (1980). Selection criteria for outpatient group psychotherapy. *Hospital and Community Psychiatry, 31* (4), 245–250.

Friedman, A. S. (1975). Interaction of drug therapy with marital therapy in depressive patients. *Archives of General Psychiatry, 32,* 619–637.

Garfield, S. L., & Bergin, A. E. (Eds.). (1978). *Handbook of psychotherapy and behavior change: An empirical analysis* (2nd ed.). New York: John Wiley and Sons.

Grunebaum, H., & Kates, W. (1977). Whom to refer to group psychotherapy. *American Journal of Psychiatry, 134* (2), 130–133.

Hersen, M., & Bellack, A. (Eds.). (1978). *Behavior therapy in the psychiatric setting.* Baltimore: The Williams and Wilkins Co.

Klerman, G. L., DiMascio, A., Weissman, M., Prusoff, B., & Paykel, E. S. (1974). Treatment of depression by drugs and psychotherapy. *American Journal of Psychiatry, 131* (2), 186–190.

Kovacs, M. (1980). The efficacy of cognitive and behavior therapies for depression. *American Journal of Psychiatry, 137* (12), 1495–1501.

Krauss, J. B., & Slavinsky, A. T. (1982). *The chronically ill psychiatric patient and the community.* Boston: Blackwell Scientific Publications, p. 194.

Luborsky, L., Singer, B., & Luborsky, L. (1975, August). Comparative studies in psychotherapies. Is it true that, "Everyone has won and all must have prizes?" *Archives of General Psychiatry, 32,* 995–1008.

McLean, P. D., & Hakstian, A. R. (1979). Clinical depression: Comparative efficacy of out-patient treatments. *Journal of Consulting and Clinical Psychology, 47* (5), 818–836.

Naparstek, A. J., and Haskell, C. D. (1977) "Neighborhood approaches to mental health services''. In *Neighborhood Psychiatry*, ed. by L. B. Macht, et. al. Lexington, Mass; Lexington Books, pp. 31–42.

Orlinsky, D. E., & Howard, K. I. (1978). The relation of process to outcome in psychotherapy. In S. L. Garfield & A. E. Bergin (Eds.), *Handbook of psychotherapy and behavior change. An empirical analysis* (2nd ed.). New York: John Wiley and Sons.

Paolino, Thomas J. (1981). *Psychoanalytic psychotherapy*. New York: Brunner/Mazel Publishers.

Raunsaville, B. J., Klerman, G. L., & Weissman, M. M. (1981). Do psychotherapy and pharmacotherapy for depression conflict? *Archives of General Psychiatry, 38,* 24–29.

Rehm, L. P., Fuchs, C. Z., Roth, D. M., Kornblith, S. R., & Romano, J. M. (1979). A comparison of self-control and assertion skills treatments of depression, *Behavior Therapy, 10,* 429–442.

Rush, A. J., Beck, A. T., Kovacs, M., & Hollon, S. (1977). Comparative efficacy of cognitive therapy and pharmacotherapy in the treatment of depressed outpatients. *Cognitive Therapy and Research, 1,* 17–37.

Rush, John A. and Watkins, John T. Cognitive Therapy with psychologically naive depressed outpatients. Ed. by Emery, Gary, Hollon, Steven D. and Bedrasian, Richard C. (1981). *New Directions in Cognitive Therapy*, New York: The Guilford Press.

Sanchez, V. C., Lewinsohn, P. M., & Larson, D. W. (1980, April). Assertion training: Effectiveness in the treatment of depression. *Journal of Clinical Psychology, 36,* (2), 526–529.

Shaw, B. F. (1977). Comparison of cognitive therapy and behavior therapy in the treatment of depression. *Journal of Consulting and Clinical Psychology, 45* (4), 543–551.

Smith, M. (1982). What research says about the effectiveness of psychotherapy. *Hospital and Community Psychiatry, 33* (6), 457–461.

Smith, M., Glass, G. V., & Miller, T. I. (1980). *The benefits of psychotherapy*. Baltimore: The Johns Hopkins University Press.

Stuart, Gail Wiscarz and Sundeen, Sandra J. (1983). *Principles and Practice of Psychiatric Nursing.* 2nd ed., St. Louis, MO.: C. V. Mosby Co.

Taylor, F. G., & Marshal, W. L. (1977). Experimental analysis of a cognitive-behavioral therapy for depression. *Cognitive Therapy and Research, 1,* 59–72.

Weinstein, M. C., & Fineberg, H. V. (1980). *Clinical decision analysis*. Philadelphia: W. B. Saunders and Company, p. 3.

Weissman, M. M. (1979). The psychological treatment of depression. Evidence for the efficacy of psychotherapy alone, in comparison with, and in combination with pharmacotherapy. *Archives of General Psychiatry, 36,* 1261–1269.

Weissman, M. M., & Kasl, S. V. (1976). Help-seeking in depressed out-patients following maintenance therapy. *British Journal of Psychiatry, 129,* 252–260.

Weissman, M., & Klerman, G. L. (1977). The chronic depressive in the community: Unrecognized and poorly treated. *Comprehensive Psychiatry, 18* (6), 523–532.

Weissman, M., Prusoff, B. A., DiMascio, A., Neu, C., Goklaney, M., & Klerman, G. L. (1979). The efficacy of drugs and psychotherapy in the treatment of acute depressive episodes. *American Journal of Psychiatry, 136* (4B), 555–558.

Williams, Mark J. (1984). The Psychological Treatment of Depression. New York: The Free Press, A Division of Macmillan, Inc.

Wilson, Holly and Kneisl, Carol (1983). *Psychiatric Nursing.* Menlo Park, CA.: Addison-Wesley Publishing Co.

Wilson, P. H., Goldin, J. C., & Charbonneau-Powis, M. (1983). Comparative efficacy of behavioral and cognitive treatments of depression. *Cognitive Therapy and Research, 7* (2), 111–124.

Zeiss, A. M., Lewinsohn, P. M., & Munoz, R. F. (1979). Nonspecific improvement effects in depression using interpersonal skills training, pleasant activities, or cognitive training. *Journal of Consulting and Clinical Psychology, 47,* 427–439.

<table>
<tr><td rowspan="2">9</td><td>Masked Symptomatology In Childhood Depression</td></tr>
<tr><td>Dennis A. Nakanishi
Paula F. Price</td></tr>
</table>

Masked Symptomatology In Childhood Depression

9

Dennis A. Nakanishi
Paula F. Price

As mental health professionals in child psychiatric nursing, the authors have found that depression in children often goes underdiagnosed or misdiagnosed. This relatively new disorder gained acceptance in the Diagnostic and Statistical Manual III (DSM III) (American Psychiatric Association, 1980) using the adult criteria of depressive symptomatology for children.

For the psychiatric nurse to select and use the appropriate therapeutic nursing interventions, she or he must first gain sensitivity to the subtlety of the illness in childhood depression. The focus of the chapter is identification of masked and childhood depression and selected interventions for same.

A review of the literature indicates four theoretical formulations on childhood depression:

1. Childhood depression is rare or nonexistent (Finch, 1960; Rie, 1966; Rutter & Hersov, 1976).
2. Childhood depression is similar to the depression that adults experience (Bishop, 1980; Kashani, 1981b; Kovacs & Beck, 1977; Malmquist, 1971; Puig-Antich & Gittleman, 1980; Puig-Antich et al. 1978).
3. Childhood depression is masked by acting-out behaviors such as delinquent behavior, physical aggressiveness, truancy, experiencing school difficulty, psychosomatic reactions, and inappropriate expressions of anger (Carlson & Cantwell 1980; Cytryn & McKnew, 1972, 1974; Glaser, 1967; Lesse, 1979; Pearce, 1977).

NURSING INTERVENTIONS IN DEPRESSION   Copyright © 1985 by Grune & Stratton, Inc.
ISBN 0-8089-1710-2   All rights of reproduction in any form reserved.

4. Biochemical correlates of childhood depression indicate similar research findings with adult endogenous depression (Cytryn & McKnew, 1974; Kashani et al., 1981; Lewis & Lewis, 1981; McKnew & Cytryn, 1979; Poznanski et al., 1982; Shekim et al., 1977).

HISTORICAL DEVELOPMENT AND LITERATURE REVIEW

Although the earliest recognition of childhood depression occurred 200 years ago (Anthony, 1977), the paucity of documented cases and theoretical formulations, inhibited study of this disorder until the last 25 years.

The earliest papers and theoretical formulations of Jon Bowlby, Melanie Klein, Sigmund Freud, and Anna Freud explore the issues of bonding and attachment (Bowlby, 1960; Robertson & Bowlby, 1952), separation and individuation (Kernberg, 1975), grief, melancholy, and object loss (Freud, A., 1944; Freud, S. 1968). Bowlby (1960) stressed the ways in which the interplay of bonding and attachment and object loss could lead to a depressive state manifested in a child's behavior. Anna and Sigmund Freud wrote extensively on the process and results of grief and mourning as well as the differentiation between the two.

Spitz (1946) identified anaclitic depression—a behavioral response found in infants separated from their mothers after 6 months of age who previously had a normal relationship. He showed how the infant could exhibit depressive behaviors after prolonged separation from the mother. Similar findings were reported by Robertson and Bowlby in 1952.

Finch (1960) and Rie (1966) argued that childhood depression could not exist because children lack a well-developed and internalized super ego. They pointed out that as a child develops, the super ego has to grow and internalize to its final form as the mediator between the id and ego. Since a child possesses an immature developing superego, childhood depression cannot exist or, if it does exist, is rare in frequency and may be due primarily to severe grief, or mourning, or both. The psychoanalytic theorists also emphasized the role of object loss in the development of depression. They noted that depression occurs after an object loss or a symbolic object loss with the person experiencing ambivalent feelings towards the object (i.e., identification). Then the child turns the angry feelings inwards, thus experiencing depression.

Toolan noted the presence of depressive equivalents in children and how developmentally depressive feelings are expressed through a child's behavior. In 1967, Glasser spoke of the symptoms of masked childhood depression, which included school phobias, school failure (under-achievement), antisocial behavior, psychosomatic complaints, and hyperkineses.

During the 1970's child mental health professionals developed the view that childhood depression exists as a clinical entity (Bemporad & Wilson, 1978). The next logical evolvement was how to diagnose and classify childhood depression. Along with this movement came the inevitable conflicts of what guidelines should be used to diagnose and classify (Cantwell & Carlson, 1979; Cytryn & McKnew, 1972). In the late 1970s and early 1980s a general trend appeared in the DSM-III and other research articles to use adult criteria to classify childhood depression (American Psychiatric Association, 1980; Puig-Antich, 1982). In 1980, the DSM-III officially accepted the use of adult criteria to diagnose childhood depression. A decision was made not to provide a classification of masked depression in the DSM-III (Cytryn et al., 1980) because it was found not to be as useful as using the two categories, acute and chronic. In the author's view, masked childhood depression exists as evidenced by the frequency of observed behaviors seen in our clinical experience. If used in conjunction with the DSM-III criteria, the symptoms of masked childhood depression can be "unmasked" (Carlson & Cantwell, 1980), revealing a co-existing depressive disorder with a behavior disorder, such as aggressive behavior, hyperactivity, and antisocial behavior.

BIOCHEMICAL CORRELATES OF CHILDHOOD AFFECTIVE DISORDERS

There is minimal research regarding biochemical correlates of depression available in the area of childhood affective disorders. Efforts by Cytryn and McKnew (1974), Cytryn (1979), and Puig-Antich et al., (1978) have laid the foundation for continued research in this field. A focus of the studies is to test the hypothesis: Is the catecholamine metabolism similar in children as in adults?

Cytryn et al., (1974) compared levels of norepinephrine (NE) and urinary metabolites, specifically 3-methoxy-4-hydroxpheny-glyol (MHPG) and vanilly-mandelic acid (VMH), of 8 diagnosed cases of depression in children 6–12 years old with a control group of 22 normal 10-year-olds. When the data were compared, decreased levels of norepinephrine and VMH appeared in the depressed children. The investigators also found deviations in MHPG levels but not in a specific direction. Their conclusions suggested that urinary metabolites are excreted by depressed children. Changes in children with chronic-type depression seem clear-cut as opposed to masked or acute depressions.

Five years later (1979), McKnew and Cytryn continued research on the metabolites NE, VMH, and MHPG in an attempt to further clarify the previous findings. Once again they found that 9 depressed children aged 6–12 years excreted less MHPG than the control group of 22 ten-year-olds. Also, the decreased level of NE was present, thus suggesting biochemical abnormality. This finding was significant in that it suggests an important connection between biochemical abnormalities and childhood depression. Further, well-designed experiments are needed to provide additional data and results.

A pilot study by Puig-Antich et al. (1978) identified a major depressive disorder in 13 prepubertal children, as diagnosed by the research diagnostic criteria, who were later treated with imipramine. This suggested the possibility that prepubertal and adult major depressive disorders are basically the same illness. In addition, the fact that the 13 children responded to a trial of imipramine implies a biochemical factor in childhood depression.

The suggestion that children can have an endogenous depression similar neuroendocrinologically to an adult endogenous depression led to a study by Poznanski et al., (1982) in which 18 dysphoric children were tested with the dexamethasome suppression test (DST).

In this study, 6–12 year-old children received 0.5 mg Dexamethasome at 11 p.m.; at 4 p.m. the next day, a blood level was drawn. All home and school activity was to have remained the same during the day. Results similar to those found in plasma levels of depressed adults indicate a neuroendocrinologically similarity between adults and children's endogenous depression.

MASKED DEPRESSION IN CHILDREN

Cytryn and McKnew (1974) defined a masked depression reaction as one in which "the depression does not manifest itself in a clearly recognizable form, but rather the child may show a variety of primary emotional disorders including hyperactivity, aggressive behavior, psychosomatic illness, hypochondriasis, and delinquency. The underlying depression is inferred by the presence of depressive fantasy material and periodic displays of overt depressive affect."

The early works of Toolan (1962), and Glaser (1967), led to the theoretical formulation of masked depression in childhood. Their observations of masked childhood depression indicate that the child's behavioral symptoms not usually associated with depression (Lachenmeyer, 1982) such as truancy, school phobia, psychosomatic illness, delinquency, hyperactivity, over-aggressive behavior, temper tantrums, and disobedience, "mask" a depression instead of verbalizing a depressive episode. He noted how a child with depressive feelings will displace those feelings with the above mentioned behaviors (Kovacs & Beck, 1977). The acting-out of these feelings further decrease the child's self esteem. These behaviors should be viewed as evidence of depression. Glaser's concept includes the additional features of "depressive elements" as negative self-evaluation and feelings of rejection. Depression, he points out, is manifested in three areas: (1) behavior problems, i.e., disobedience and truancy; (2) psychosomatic reactions, i.e., school phobia; and (3) psychophysiologic reactions (Kovacs & Beck, 1977).

A decade after Toolan's and Glaser's work, Cytryn and McKnew (1972) classified childhood depression in three categories: masked, acute, and chronic, with masked childhood depression occurring most frequently. From their work emerged a study regarding childhood defense mechanisms. They found that "a hierarchy of defense systems existed which was progressively less capable of protecting the children against depression" (Cytryn & McKnew, 1972). The results showed that children diagnosed with masked depressive reactions exhibited anger more openly than the other two categories and their fantasy themes were filled with aggression, violence, death, and low self-esteem.

The depressive process in children manifests itself in three different ways (Cytryn & McKnew, 1974): (1) fantasy—depressive themes, elicited by dreams, play, or projective tests, in children's fantasy include abandonment, death, suicide, object loss, blame, and mistreatment; (2) verbal expression—if the child speaks of themes of hopelessness, helplessness, being unloved, suicidal ideation, guilt, or body-image issues; (3) mood behavior—if a clinician can observe and/or collect data for behavioral changes in sleep, appetite, body posture, or behavioral symptoms associated with masked depression.

With this information, Cytryn and McKnew observed that three levels of defenses exist for depressed children to either avoid dealing with or expressing the depression (Cytryn & McKnew, 1974).

- 1st level   Use of denial, acting out, avoidance, splitting, and projection or introjection as defense mechanisms, or both.
- 2nd level   Use of dissociation of affect and reaction formation.
- 3rd level   All of the defenses fail against the depressive illness.

In the 1970s, clinical interests in this disorder intensified (Bramberg, 1973; Kovacs & Beck, 1977; Malinquist, 1977; Poznanski, 1970, 1980, 1981; and Puig-Antich, et al., 1978). By 1980, Cytryn et al. spoke of reassessing their diagnoses of masked childhood depression by adult criteria. That same year Carlson and Cantwell (1980) showed the use of standard evaluation tools with systematic interviews and adult diagnostic criteria. Their findings concluded that if the behavioral symptoms of masked childhood depression are present, the clinician should be aware that depression may be overshadowed. If the clinician conducts a systematic interview the depression will surface. Also, if the presence of masked childhood depressive symptomatolgy exists, then the clinician should throughly assess for a depressive reaction.

The following case example provides a representative picture of a child experiencing masked childhood depression.

Dusty, a 7-year-old male, was admitted to a children's day hospital for the following behavioral problems: physically hitting other children, swearing, spitting, defiant and oppositional behaviors, severe temper tantrums, and separation anxiety. Due to school failure he had to repeat kindergarten.

A full scale psychological testing battery showed Dusty's IQ to be 125 verbal and 94 performance, indicating some form of perceptual motor dysfunction. Personality testing

(TAT and Rorschach), along with behavioral observations, revealed a child who was affectively dominated. Personality testing also indicated unfulfilled interpersonal transaction as well as violent and unsatisfactory outcomes coupled with a high level of emotionality. His potential for aggressive acting-out was high and predictable.

During the course of his stay, Dusty's parents experienced marital problems, undergoing a trial separation followed by divorce. Both at home and school, he became increasingly disruptive with temper tantrums. He struck and verbally abused his peers and staff members. As the acting-out behavior escalated, he had an increasing difficulty verbalizing his feelings. Only after an incident, in which his mother had to physically restrain Dusty from hitting his head on the floor, was he able to verbalize his feelings. Frustrated and angry, he continually assaulted his peers physically, creating a disruptive atmosphere in the classroom as well as alienating himself from everyone. Toward the end of his stay, Dusty complained of feeling bad and started to experience stomach aches.

Dusty's case provides a picture of masked childhood depression characterized by acting-out, school failure, physical aggressiveness, and delinquent behavior, along with psychosomatic complaints.

The detection of childhood depression requires a thorough psychosocial assessment, including school and peer relationships, behavioral and affective observation, projective testing, and if warranted, laboratory testing for biological diagnostic markers for depression. Treatment consists of psychosocial interventions, such as milieu play, individual and group modalities, and parent or family therapy, or both. The various modalities assist the child in alleviating the underlying depression and modifying the acting-out behavior.

Aggressive and antisocial behavior are signs of depression in children, since they tend to express their hostilities inwardly toward themselves, or toward those who threaten their psychological well-being. A therapeutic milieu will provide the emotionally labile child with a sense of well-being and safety by providing external controls which reassures the child that he will not be allowed to hurt self or others when a loss of control occurs.

THERAPEUTIC MILIEU

A therapeutic milieu anticipates events and emotions that internally precede behavioral outbursts. Identifying and verbalizing these factors for the child assists in reality orientation and defusing the situation. Redl's 1952 concept of life-space interviewing can be utilized to modify acting-out behaviors and increase verbalization of the problem. This concept assists in reality testing for children who misinterpret interpersonal events and helps the child to recognize that maladaptive behavior results in negative responses.

Life-space interviewing provides for a nonjudgmental interaction. Confronted with the inappropriate behavior, the child is asked to discuss the precipitating events. The event is then discussed to evaluate the response with other alternatives that could be employed. The following example illustrates the technique used following an incident in which a child climbed on monkey bars during recess and purposely pulled another youngster off the bars.

Therapist:	Perhaps you could tell me what happened here?
Child:	I didn't do anything!
Therapist:	Let me tell you what I saw. You were playing on the monkey bars with J. and you suddenly pulled him off.
Child:	It wasn't my fault! He started it!
Therapist:	J. started it?
Child:	Yes, he was standing on my hand!
Therapist:	Do you feel he was standing on your hand on purpose?
Child:	Yes, he was coming down and saw me there.
Therapist:	Is it difficult to see below you when you go down backwards?
Child:	I think he did it on purpose.
Therapist:	But do you really know that's what J. was doing?
Child:	Yes, he . . . .
Therapist:	I realize you were upset and hurting, but what else could you have done?
Child:	I don't know.
Therapist:	Think about it—what else could you have done and not get time-out?*
Child:	I could have told you.
Therapist:	Or?
Child:	I could have told him to get off my hand.
Therapist:	Right! Why don't you try it out next time and in that way you won't miss any of the fun. Go on and play.
Child:	Ok.

Use of this type of intervention after an acting-out incident must be performed consistently. Ultimately, the child will learn that more appropriate action exists that bring positive results. The life-space interviewing concept also assists the child in decreasing accumulation of hostilities or frustrations, provides emotional support, reiterates expectations, and maintains a relationship with the child to prevent withdrawal from others.

Another intervention utilized for creating a therapeutic milieu is the concept of time-out. This is an intervention that consists of removing the child from all sources of reinforcement or stimulation immediately after the inappropriate behavior has occurred. It is a brief period of time of from 2–10 minutes. According to Erickson (1982) time-out should not be viewed as a method to frighten the

---

*Time-out: removing child from all sources of reinforcement or stimulation immediately after an inappropriate behavior has occured.

child. At home, the child might be placed in a room that contains no toys, TV, or radios. At school, the child might be removed to the hallway or enter a time-out room that is well lit. If the hallway is used, staff and other children must be informed that no attention should be given to the child until the period of time-out is completed. Time-out rooms are usually employed for serious acting-out or loss of control. It is important that all children in the setting have the opportunity to view the room, and that clear delineation of the types of inappropriate behaviors that will illicit the use of time-out be explained. After time-out is used, a brief discussion occurs during which the behavior is once again identified and the consequences are reiterated.

Another method of creating the milieu and decreasing aggressive and/or antisocial behavior is that of response cost. This involves the removal of a positive reinforcer immediately after the occurrence of the inappropriate behavior. Examples of this would include removing of a favorite toy or exclusion from a special field trip.

Substantial positive changes in behavior have occurred by introducing positive reinforcement that increases appropriate behavior by contingent acquiring and decreases inappropriate behavior by consequential withdrawal. Giving points to a child for making it through recess without fighting, or completing an assignment without cursing in the classroom, can be applied toward a special outing. When the inappropriate behavior occurs, a predetermined number of points are withdrawn.

Another example of cost response is the token economy. Erickson (1982) believes that "token economies" are aimed at providing positive reinforcement for appropriate behaviors. As with the point system, the cost response for each inappropriate display of behavior is determined prior to initiation of the intervention, and is presented to the child.

Structuring the milieu and applying techniques of life space interviewing, not only decreases inappropriate behavior and shapes appropriate response but also assist in developing the therapeutic alliance necessary for other psychotherapeutic approaches. Such an alliance is important to the success of compliance with individual and group therapy, as well as making positive changes in behavior.

INDIVIDUAL AND GROUP PSYCHOTHERAPY

According to Nelms and Brady (1980) individual and group therapy is most widely used for the treatment of depression in children. "The nurse's role in therapy is based on his or her clinical expertise. . . ." Depending on the nurses' theoretical focus, the techniques and approaches may differ. The goal is to assist the child to cope with his current life difficulties.

Play and individual therapies are modalities most often used with school age children. Axline (1969) states that play therapy "is an opportunity for the child to play out his feelings and problems. . . ." During play therapy, the emotional content underlying conflicts and impulses is interpreted to the child. The therapist must provide an atmosphere that is free of threat and communicates concern and interest.

When play therapy begins, the therapist can use a combination of active participation and nondirective therapy. Active participation may appear in the form of warm acceptance of the child's activities and verbalization, joining in if the child requests the participation and reflecting what the child appears to be feeling. In nondirective therapy (Axline, 1969), the therapist recognizes feelings and reflects them back to the child, who, in turn, should develop insight into behavior.

During the first psychotherapy sessions, the therapist should establish several basic expectations. Since therapy usually occurs in the therapist's office, the creation of a safe environment is important. The guidelines would include that the child does not physically abuse the therapist or the furnishings within the office, and should be allowed to choose whatever toy or game needed to express feelings.

Finally, the two major goals for psychotherapy of the depressed child are (1) the establishment of adaptive controls and defenses by providing encouragement to verbalize anger or express it symbolically through play and use of acceptable activities and age-appropriate games to modify and inhibit the aggression and acting-out behavior; and (2) the improvement of self-esteem. The integration of play and discussion assists the child in exploring his or her concept of self. The therapist highlights and develops his or her positive qualities and assists in working through self-blame and feelings of punishment. Self-esteem slowly improves with exposure to the climate of warmth and acceptance generated by the therapist. Garfinkel and Golombek (1972) notes that developing an honest and nonjudgmental relationship aids the child in developing appropriate skills for relieving unwanted feelings and behavior. Soon the child focuses on the here and now and the therapist emphasizes the developmental tasks that the child needs to work out.

GROUP THERAPY

Group therapy serves as an adjunct to play and individual therapy modalities. Ginott (1975) observes that group is the "treatment of choice for children aged three to nine." Since acting-out behavior tends to inappropriately dissapate the depressive/aggressive feelings in the child, group therapy becomes an appropriate approach for the child. Group therapy is based on the belief that the acting-out depressed child has the need to be accepted by peers (an age-appropriate developmental task for a school-age child), and that modifying impulses and changing behavior are revisions to be made to assure acceptance.

In addition to acting-out behavior, the depressed child typically exercises fewer social skills. Group therapy is an appropriate vehicle for social skills training. Feedback in the form of verbal and nonverbal peer interaction plays an important educational goal. Depressed children typically demonstrate behavior traits such as temper tantrums, physical aggressiveness, and ignoring the rights and wishes of others. In addition, they tease and embarrass others, and demand immediate gratification of their wishes. In a group setting, these children can learn how to express their feelings, defend their rights, and interact in a more adaptive and socially appropriate manner.

During group time, the members are directed in the use of peer pressure to modify unacceptable behavior. Congruent communication should be used to point out the behavior and assist children in developing more appropriate coping mechanisms and social skills. The therapist gives positive reinforcement and serves as a model of self-control. The therapist also interprets the children's behavior, encouraging them to express their problems and anxieties to each other. Group therapy provides the opportunity to develop insight into the reasons for behavior, helping children to acquire more appropriate skills in the area of peer interaction and decreased feelings of frustration. Using play material also encourages activities that reflect conflict, such as playing with dolls that help to decrease fears of abandonment and jealousy of a new sibling, or playing house to demonstrate safety and consistency to children from chaotic homes.

Ginott (1975) states that the end result of group therapy is "a strengthened ego, a modified superego and an enhanced self-image." Changes in behavior should occur partially because self-knowledge develops through relationships with others; and the child must confront the behavior due to peer response. The child must use the group when facing the problem and the situation provoking it. The following excerpt demonstrates an interaction from a group session that involves teaching the use of peer pressure and how to develop more appropriate social skills for a particularily aggressive child. During this session, a group of five children were building a tower from cardboard boxes. The child in question became frustrated when his demanding suggestions were not accepted by the other children.

J.: (yelling) I told you to do it this way (the child proceeds to yank blocks from the others).

P. & S.: No—we decided to do it this way (whiney tone of voice and pulling on blocks).

J.: Ok (proceeds to kick down tower).
Group looks to therapist, complaining:

Therapist: I wonder how the group feels about what just happened?

P.:	I'm going to get you (heads for J.).
Therapist:	P., do you remember what happens if you hit during group?
P.:	But he . . . .
Therapist:	What can you do instead of hitting?
P.:	Tell him I'm mad.
S.:	I don't want him to play with us.
J.:	You weren't letting me play anyway.
Therapist:	You felt left out?
J.:	Yes.
Therapist:	What could have been done instead of kicking the tower down?
J.:	I could have shown them it would work.
Therapist:	(to group) What do you think? Does it make sense to let each other demonstrate things to see if it works?
Group:	He never listens—it would fall down.
Therapist:	Could you start again after J. sees it doesn't work?
Group:	Guess so.
Therapist:	How does the group want to handle J. if he does something similar again?
Group:	Give him time-out once and if he does it again he can't play for the rest of the group.
Therapist:	How about it J.? Does that seem fair?
J.:	Yes—I guess.

From this interaction, the children learn more appropriate ways to express their feelings and how to compromise and channel frustration into more socially acceptable expressions. The children learn to sublimate aggressive acting-out behavior in a more appropriate way. Meaningful interactions with other children are provided through activities and situations existing in the group environment. The opportunity exists for competitive games and for expression of repressed hostility.

FAMILY THERAPY

The participation of the parent or family in the therapeutic process is included in the treatment used for the acting-out depressed child. The nature of family interactions is explored in addition to assisting the parent or family in coping with and minimizing the behavior. According to Toolan (1977), parents need to be actively involved in the therapeutic process . . . "this procedure is based on the assumption that the child's pathology often arises from the parent's inability to relate to their children". Often feeling guilty or embarrassed by the child's behavior, parents readily deny the existence of any problems. Conjunct therapy will assist the therapist in understanding the interaction and relationship between the parents and the child. The process becomes helpful to understanding and altering family dynamics.

During family sessions, the therapist must provide an atmosphere that encourages open and free communication. Through such an environment, the therapist can ascertain the relationships in the home, which will assist in determining ways the family supports the child's problem. David, a child with difficulty in controlling impulses, did not respond well to limit setting; he constantly tested limits. During the first family session, part of the problem became obvious: David attempted to distract the adults and become the center of attention. The parents allowed the behavior to continue with minimal limit-setting and with no consistency. After several minutes, the therapist acted as a role model for the parents and firmly limited the child's behavior by confronting and limiting any inappropriate attention seeking behavior. The parents were amazed; the therapist then pointed out that a child needs to know the expectations of adults, what the limits are, and consistency of consequential intervention. The therapist further explained that if the child doesn't experience consistency he or she does not feel safe or feels a lack of caring, and proceeds to act-out these feelings in an inappropriate manner.

To a large extent, family therapy focuses on reality factors in child rearing, such as discipline and specific fears. Satir (1964) points out that the family needs to be assisted in learning to recognize and accept individual differences. The parents are taught to realize that differences should be used positively and to communicate feelings.

A common problem is lack of consistency, expectations, and limits of the child's behavior between the two parents. As a result the child learns how to manipulate the parents and increase inappropriate behavior to meet his needs.

Another approach to family therapy is the systems intervention concept (Minuchin, 1974). The child no longer becomes the only focus, and the entire family is considered a psychosocial system. Minuchin (1974) assumes that the child's problem reflects the maintenance of the family's balance. In other words, if the child's problem disappears, the family will soon develop new problems or the family system will not remain intact. Therefore, all interactions must be considered, including marital discord, the child's views of parents and siblings, and the child's view of him- or herself within the system. David, the child mentioned earlier, had learned to manipulate his parents during their frequent separations in order to decrease his anxieties regarding abandonment and lack of love. He used antisocial, aggressive behavior to gain attention from others. The parents were instructed in ways to increase their communication skills, thereby becoming aware of David's manipulation. They began to demonstrate a united front regarding limits and developed a consistent approach. When David began to act-out during mealtime they gave a warning of the consequence. When the behavior occurred, he was removed to the kitchen regardless of his plea not to repeat the behavior.

Parents need to recognize that it is behavior, not the child, that is unacceptable. In addition, they must inform the child that once the consequence for inappropriate behavior has occurred, the incident and anger are over, and the child begins with a clean slate. It is often helpful for parents to have group therapy with other parents. Such a mechanism provides mutual support and creates an avenue for expression of concerns and fears, and for comparing effective interventions. This approach helps parents to see that they are not alone in their problems and to foster self esteem.

PSYCHOPHARMACOLOGY

The final therapeutic mode used in the treatment of childhood depression is psychopharmacology. When the depressive symptomatology of the child does not remit with psychotherapy, and he continues to have difficulty functioning at home, with peers, and at school, medication is recommended. According to Kashani et al. (1981b), antidepressants have been used for children since 1962. If drugs are used, comprehensive approaches mentioned in earlier sections also continue.

The tricyclics group represents the most commonly prescribed medication for childhood depression with imipramine used most often. After the proper dosage has been titrated, the child should respond in 2–3 weeks, with remission evident in 6–8 weeks. A major advantage of antidepressants is that they produce an effect in a relatively short time. Pearce (1980–81) considers this important "since any interruption to steady maturation and development can have serious consequences."

Side effects include atropine-like effects, dryness of the mouth, and drowsiness. The clinician reassures the parents and child that these symptoms are temporary and to suggest ways for decreasing these effects, such as giving the child some sugarless hard candy for mouth dryness. Dizziness, tremors, sweating, nausea, and anorexia also can occur. After remission of depressive symptoms, the drug should be gradually withdrawn since symptoms of tension, insomnia, nausea, and headaches may appear. The child needs to be monitored closely and to communicate with parents regarding side effects.

There are several considerations to observe prior to initiating drug therapy. The act of prescribing a drug implies that the depression is not the responsibility of the child nor the parents, and they may not actively work to make appropriate changes. Further concerns regarding drug interactions and accidental drug ingestion, or abuse, or both. A tendency to look to the drug for help rather than developing more appropriate coping skills or resolving problems will occur unless specific interventions are combined with drug therapy. Parental cooperation is essential when initiating drug therapy on the child. A simple but thorough explanation of the mechanism of antidepressants in relation to depression is mandatory. The parents are responsible for administration and safe-keeping of all medications. They should be encouraged to take an active role in planning how the drug will be given, as well the route and schedule. These approaches aid in gaining parental and child compliance to the treatment process.

SPECIFIC INTERVENTIONS

This section will deal with specific interventions of the therapist targeted for decreasing antisocial, aggressive, and manipulative behavior, as well as increasing self-esteem in the depressed child.

Manipulative Behaviors

• *Try not to argue with the child.* As an alternative response offer recognition for the feelings the child expresses and voice an understanding of the situation described.

• *Reestablish with the child both the situation and immediate problem.* Make expectations clear, and reinforce that the child must deal with you.

• *Do not discuss other staff/parents who are not present.* Encourage the child to bring complaints to the person with whom he or she had problems. Suggest a meeting of all those involved to straighten out a misunderstanding.

• *Keep communication lines open.* This prevents the child from splitting adults or staff. These particular children can sound convincing and introduce confusion.

• *Be empathic with the child.* Recognize that he or she seems to be in a real predicament. Let the child know, however, that you cannot sort out a situation if you were not there.

• *Integrate the child into appropriate milieu activity when he or she is calm.*

Aggression

• *Anticipate a triggering event for the child and verbalize the behavior whenever possible.* Examples of triggering events are: (1) narcissistic injuries of all sorts, or an anticipation of same; (2) feelings of separatism or abandonment, or an anticipation of same; (3) fantasizing fear of injury from others; (4) experiences of powerlessness and helplessness; and (5) warding off of the depressive affect.

• *Anticipate triggering emotions that internally precede behavioral out-burst and empathically verbalize the identified feelings to the child.*

• *Reward with praise any evidence that the child demonstrates any indepen-dent mastery of aggressive impulses.*

• *Control explosive and temper out-bursts.*   Give the child an opportunity to calm down with one-to-one discussion in classroom. If the above does not help, remove the child from the classroom for the least restrictive amount of time. Foster the child's participation in regaining control of self. If that does not help, remove the child to a time-out area for the least amount of time necessary. Reward the child for gaining control.

• *Help the child to conceptualize the problem.*   Do this during the free time as a "project" to work on and encourage verbalization of the child's thoughts on resolving his or her problems.

• *Reward Verbalization of emotions and thoughts.*   This can be done as a means of handling aggression.

• *Maintain firm consistent limit setting.*

Hyperactivity with or without Attention-Deficit Disorder

• *Maintain child's self-esteem.*   This can be done through verbal rewarding reinforcement when appropriate.

• *Distinguish for the child the confusion of "bad self from bad and undesir-able behavior."*

• *Empathically understand the child's difficulty with impulse-self control.*

• *Form working alliance with the child.*   Utilize this on the target project and reward any success resulting from child's efforts.

• *Provide nondistracting sitting.*   This will enable you to help the child screen out stimuli.

• *Maintain proximity to adult in unstructured visually stimulating settings.*

• *Identify and discuss with the child emotional or environmental stressors that aggravate the child's underlying hyperactivity problem.*

Emotional Lability

• *Assurance.*   Assure that the child has controls of his or her own (if he or she has) and that you will help the child use those controls.

• *External control.*   Provide external control when the child's inner control doesn't hold. This may include physical holding or restraint.

• *Reassurance*   Give reassurance that the child will not be allowed to hurt him- or herself or anyone else while out of control. Praise the child when control is regained.

Poor Group Play and Uncooperativeness

- *Short attention span*   If the child has a short attention span, the interventions are to limit and redirect. If the child tunes out rules or preparation, intervene by increasing contact with various parts of group activity. If the child starts side-games, or engages another child in conversation, interventions include using group members to motivate the child's attention, and participation to reflect child's behavior back to the self. If the child loses interest or drifts off, the intervention is to increase the child's awareness of his or her role, and others' feelings.

- *Refusal to play by the rules.*   When the child does not play by the rules, limits, or boundaries of activities, intervene by assessing the problem. It may be lack of skill, fear, or competitiveness. Teach skills. Limit and control the disruption of the group. Use the group members to increase "empathy" and self-observation.

- *Afraid to try an activity.*   If the child is afraid to try activity and either doesn't begin, or withdraws from it, intervention can include teaching the skills of the game to increase self-confidence; allowing the child to observe or participate on the edge; giving special "graded" positions in the game, starting with the least demanding role; and giving incentive to the group to include the child.

- *Excessive competitiveness.*   When a child is excessively competitive, interventions include limiting and controlling. If the child cannot take turns, intervention will be use of empathy to increase trust. If the child has a "must win" attitude or is overly aggressive, interventions include "Interpreting" to prepare the child for the game, increasing cognitive mediation, and delay of impulses. When the child cannot accept loss, the interventions are to "talk the child through" experiences, and have the child verbally rehearse requirements of his or her behavior. The group can discuss winning and losing.

CONCLUSION

The frequency of occurrence of childhood depression, especially masked childhood depression, is widely underestimated. It is also underdiagnosed or misdiagnosed. As a child develops, he or she experiences various psychosocial stressors, such as school performance, divorce in the home, peer pressure, and others. If the child has underdeveloped or overstressed coping mechanisms, he or she becomes at high risk for a depressive illness.

The clinician should be aware of the DSM-III criteria for childhood depression and, as these authors suggest, be cognizant of the masked depressive symptomatology: hyperactive behavior, physically acting-out, psychosomatic illness, hypochondriasis, delinquent behavior, failure in school performance, and disobedient or oppositional behavior, or both. If masked depressive symptomatolgy is present as a complaint, the clinician should consider the possible occurrence of a childhood depressive illness.

The nurse has the opportunity to apply research and/or treatment plans not only to the psychiatric setting but to the pediatric floor as well. A need exists for longitudinal treatment-outcome studies in addition to the biochemical research now in its infancy stage. Recognition of these research needs should be emphasized to the potential researcher because of the complexity of research in children due to the developmental stages. The psychiatric nurse can provide profound insight, develop better treatment interventions, and increase the amount of research into childhood depression.

REFERENCES

American Psychiatric Association. (1980). *Diagnostic and statistical manual of mental disorders* (3rd ed.). Washington, D.C.: American Psychiatric Association.

Anthony, E. J. (1977). Depression in children. In G. D. Burrows (Ed.), *Handbook of studies on depression*. New York: Excerpta Medica.

Axline, V. M. (1969). *Play therapy* (p. 9). New York: Balantine.

Bemporad, J., & Wilson, A. (1978). A developmental approach to depression in childhood and adolescence. *Journal of the American Academy of Psychoanalysis, 6*(3), 325–352.

Bishop, F. (1980). Depression in childhood. *Australian Family Physician, 9*, 333–336.

Bowlby, J. (1960). Childhood mourning and its implication for psychiatry. *American Journal of Psychiatry, 118*, 481–498.

Cantwell, D. P., & Carlson, G. A. (1979). Problems and prospects in the study of childhood depression. *Journal of Nervous and Mental Disease, 167*, 522–529.

Carlson, G. A., & Cantwell, D. P. (1980). Unmasking masked depression in children and adolescents. *American Journal of Psychiatry, 137*(4), 445–449.

Cytryn, L. (1979). Current research in childhood depression. *Journal of the American Academy of Child Psychiatry, 3*, 583, 585.

Cytryn, L., & McKnew, D. H. (1972). Proposed classification of childhood depression. *American Journal of Psychiatry, 129*, 149–155.

Cytryn, L., & McKnew, D. H. (1974). Factors influencing the changing clinical expression of the depressive process in children. *American Journal of Psychiatry, 131*(8), 879–881.

Cytryn, L., McKnew, D. H., & Bunney, W. (1980). Diagnosis of depression in children: A reassessment. *American Journal of Psychiatry, 137*, 22–25.

Cytryn, L., McKnew, D. H., Logue, M., & Desai, R. B. (1974). Biochemical correlates of affective disorders in children. *Archives of General Psychiatry, 31*, 659–661.

Erickson, M. T. (1982). Treatment: The psychotherapies and pharmacotherapy. In M. T. Erickson (Ed.), *Child Psychotherapy*. New York: Prentice Hall, p. 134.

Finch, S. M. (1960). *Fundamentals of child psychiatry*. New York: W. W. Norton.

Freud, A., & Burlingham, D. (1944). *Infants without families*. New York: International Universities.

Freud, S. (1968). Mourning and melancholia: The meaning of despair. In W. Gaylin (Ed.), *Psychoanalytic contributions to the Understanding of Depression*. New York: Science House.

Garfinkel, B. and Golombek, H. (1972). Suicide and depression in childhood and adolescence. In *Common syndromes in child psychiatry* (pp. 151–164). New York: Prentice Hall.

Ginott, H. G. (1975). Group therapy with children. In G. M. Gazda (Ed.), *Basic approaches to group psychotherapy and group counseling*. Springfield, Ill.: Thomas.

Glaser, K. (1967). Masked depression in childhood and adolescence. *American Journal of Psychiatry, 21,* 565–574.

Kashani, J., Barbero, G., & Bolender, F. (1981a). Depression in hospitalized pediatric patients. *Journal of the American Academy of Child Psychiatry, 20,* 123–134.

Kashani, J. H., Husain, A., Shekim, W. O., Hodges, K. K., Cytryn, L., & McKnew, D. H. (1981b). Current perspectives on childhood depression: An overview. *American Journal of Psychiatry, 138*(2), 143–153.

Kernberg, O. F. (1975). On Melanie Klein. In A. M. Freeman, H. I. Kaplan, & B. J. Sadock (Eds.), *Comprehensive Textbook of Psychiatry*. Baltimore: Williams & Wilkins.

Kovacs, M., & Beck, A. T. (1977). An empirical-clinical approach toward a definition of childhood depression. In J. G. Schulterbrandt, & A. Raskin (Eds.), *Depression in Childhood* (pp. 1–25). New York: Raven Press.

Lachenmeyer, J. R. (1982). Specials disorders of childhood: Depression, school phobia and anorexia nervosa. In *Psychopathology in Childhood* (pp. 56). New York: Gardner Press.

Lesse, S. (1979). Behavioral problems masking depression—cultural and clinical survey. *American Journal of Psychotherapy, 35*(1), 41–53.

Lewis, M., & Lewis, D. (1981). Depression in childhood: A biopsychosocial perspective. *American Journal of Psychotherapy, 35*(3), 323–329.

Malmquist, C. P. (1971). Depression in childhood and adolescence. *The New England Journal of Medicine, 284*(16), 887–961.

Malmquist, C. P. (1977). Childhood depression: A clinical and behavioral perspective. In J. G. Schulterbrandt, & A. Raskin (Eds.), *Depression in Childhood* (pp. 33–59). New York: Raven Press.

McKnew, D. H., & Cytryn, L. (1979). Urinary metabolites in chronically depressed children. *Journal of the American Academy of Child Psychiatry, 18,* 608–615.

Minuchin, S. (1974). *Families and family therapy*. Cambridge, MA: Harvard University Press.

Nelms, B. C., & Brady, M. A. (1980, July–Aug.). Assessment and intervention: The depressed school aged child. *Pediatric Nursing,* pp. 15–19.

Pearce, J. (1977). Annotation: Depressive disorder in childhood. *Journal of Child Psychology and Psychiatry, 18,* 79–82.

Pearce, J. (1980–81). Drug treatment of depression in children. *Acta Paedopsychiatric, 46,* 317–328.

Poznanski, E., & Zrull, J. P. (1970). Childhood Depression. *Archives of General Psychiatry, 23,* 8–15.

Poznanski, E. O. (1980–81). Childhood depression: The outcome. *Acta Paedopsychiatric, 46,* 297–304.

Poznanski, E. O., Carroll, B. J., Banegas, M. C., Cook, S. C., & Grossman, J. A. (1982). The desamethasome suppression test in prepubertal depressed children. *American Journal of Psychiatry, 139*(3), 321–324.

Puig-Antich, J. (1982). The use of R.D.C. criteria for major depressive disorder in child and adolescent psychiatric patients. *Journal of the American Academy of Child Psychiatry, 21,* 291–293.

Puig-Antich, J., Blau, S., Marx, N., Greenhill, L. L., & Chambers, W. (1978). Prepubertal major depressive disorder. *Journal of the American Academy of Child Psychiatry, 17,* 695–707.

Puig-Antich, J., & Gittelman, R. (1980). Depression in childhood and adolescence. In E. S. Paykey (Ed.), *Handbook of Affective Disorders* (pp. 379–392). London: Churchill.

Redl, F. (1952). *Controls from within: Techniques for the treatment of the aggressive child.* Glencoe, Ill.: Free Press.

Rie, H. E. (1966). Depression in childhood: A survey of some pertinent contributions. *Journal of the American Academy of Child Psychiatry, 5,* 653–685.

Robertson, J., & Bowlby, J. (1952). Responses of young children to separation from their mothers. *Cour du Centre International de l'Enfance, 2,* 131–142.

Rutter, M., & Hersov, L. (1976). *Child psychiatry: Modern approaches.* London: Blackwell.

Satir, V. M. (1964). *Conjoint family therapy.* Palo Alto, Calif.: Science and Behavior.

Shekim, W. O., Dekirmenjian, H., & Chapel, J. L. (1977). Urinary catecholamine metabolites in hyperkinetic boys treated with d-amphetamine. *American Journal of Psychiatry, 134*(11), 1276–1278.

Spitz, R. (1946). Anaclitic depression. *Psychoanalytic Study of the Child, 2,* 113–117.

Toolan, J. M. (1962). Depression in children and adolescents. *American Journal of Orthopsychiatry, 32,* 404–414.

Toolan, J. M. (1977). Therapy of depressed and suicidal children. *American Journal of Psychotherapy, 31,* 2,5, 243–251.

SELECTED READINGS

Blumberg, M. (1977). Depression in children on a general pediatric service. *American Journal of Psychotherapy, 31,* 20–32.

Brumback, R. A., & Weinberg, W. A. (1977). Childhood depression: An explanation of a behavior disorder in children. *Perceptual and Motor Skills, 44,* 911–916.

Campbell, J., & Mahesh, D. (1980). Childhood depression. *The Journal of the Indiana State Medical Association,* pp. 669–673.

Cohen-Sandler, R., & Berman, A. L. (1980). Diagnosis and treatment of childhood depression and self destructive behavior. *Journal of Family Practice, 2*(11), 51–58.

Commins, S., & Husler, A. (1980). Depression in children and adolescence. *Pediatric Annals, 9*(7), 263–268.

Frame, C., Matson, J. L., Sonis, W. A., Fialkov, M. J., & Kazdin, A. E. (1982). Behavioral treatment of depression in a prepubertal child. *Journal of Behavior Therapy, 13*(3), 239–243.

Graham, J. (1980–81). Depressive disorders in children—a reconsideration. *Acta Paedospychiatric, 46,* 285–296.

Petti, T. A. (1980). Residential and inpatient treatment of children and adolescents. In G. P. Shoevard, R. M. Bensen, & B. J. Blineder (Eds.), *The Treatment of Emotional Disorders in Children and Adolescents* (pp. 209–220). New York: Spectrum.

Petti, T. A., Bornstein, M., Delamater, A., & Conners, C. K. (1980). Evaluation and multimodal treatment of a depressed prepubertal girl. *Journal of the American Academy of Child Psychiatry, 19,* 690–702.

Toolan, J. M. (1981). Depression and suicide in children: An overview. *American Journal of Psychotherapy, 35*(3), 311–322.

Welner, Z. (1978). Childhood depression: An overview. *The Journal of Nervous and Mental Disorders, 166*(1), 588–593.

10

Milieu Intervention for Mania

David Duda
Jane Ulsafer-Van Lanen

W hen the nursing report alerts the oncoming shift that a manic patient has been admitted, eyes usually roll back in staff member's heads. The report will include the manic's exhibiting behaviors: hyperactivity demonstrated by excessive talking, frequent changing of clothes, and many telephone calls—as well as the reactions of other patients on the unit—a reaction that can range from amusement to anger and fear. In their reports, however, nurses all too often fail to indicate specific nursing interventions that have been implemented to provide the therapeutic care that protects the patient's dignity and prevents milieu disruption.

One has to examine the manipulative aura that mania creates to understand why nurses frequently fail to provide effective care. Mania intensifies specific interactional abilities that allow an individual to control communication and relationships. It creates increased perceptiveness to vulnerabilities in others, increased rate and intensity of speech, and an unending supply of self-confidence and energy. These qualities allow the manic patient a certain edge when establishing relationships. Unfortunately these relationships are shallow and superficial, and soon the antics that previously entertained patients and staff now have them exhausted and angry.

This chapter will examine mania and its effect on a hospital milieu. Secondly, it will provide systematic approaches for treating the acute manic episode and the chronic manic patient. Particular focus will be given to interpersonal interventions and the nurse's role in biochemical intervention. Finally, milieu variables will be identified that can be mobilized to ensure therapeutic care for the individual patient and the remainder of the patient population.

NURSING INTERVENTIONS IN DEPRESSION   Copyright © 1985 by Grune & Stratton, Inc.
ISBN 0-8089-1710-2

MANIA

The Diagnostic and Statistical Manual of Mental Disorders (DSM-III) (American Psychiatric Association, 1980) diagnoses manic-depressive illness based on major areas such as mood, behavioral symptoms, the duration of symptoms, thought process, and ruling out organicity (e.g., drug-induced mania). Of these areas, the list of behaviors, mood, and thought processes are important to nurses because many of these symptoms are present in the hospitalized patient. The remaining criteria of DSM-III are used to differentiate manic-depressive illness from psychoses, drug-induced mania, or schizophrenia.

Seven behaviors listed in DSM-III (1980) describe the patient in a manic phase:

1. Hyperactivity.
2. Increase in volume and pressure of speech.
3. A subjective report or verbal display of flight of ideas.
4. Inflated self-esteem (overconfidence).
5. Decreased need for sleep.
6. Distractability.
7. An excessive involvement in social interactions that have a high potential for painful consequences with no insight by the patient.

Patients demonstrating these behaviors can disarm the most experienced nurse and disrupt the unit. Overconfidence and grandiosity are mental states which, when marked by an elated mood, can make an individual very powerful in relationships. Thus, manic patients often get their way because of behavior that appears as charm, wit, and verbal skill. When the confidence and grandiosity are marked by an irritable mood, the manic patient may still get his or her way because the patient quickly resorts to techniques that question the nurse's competency and self-worth. Additionally, the irritable manic seems particularly adept at involving all members of the unit in his or her various complaints or "causes." Feelings of injustice, pitting staff against patient, along with constant patient complaints of unfairness, are red flags that should alert nursing staff to look for a manic patient who is not being properly managed by medications, individual, or milieu therapy.

CLASSIFICATION OF MANIC SYMPTOMS

One analysis of the manic episode classifies it into three separate stages. This classification is very helpful in assessing the interventions needed to treat the manic patient. A longitudinal study (Carlson et al., 1973) documents behaviors manifested by the unmedicated manic patient. The assertion is made that there is a progression of symptoms that can be observed and predicted. The patient's mood, correlated with the symptoms, described in the following three sections predict the stage of mania for which staff needs to be alerted and prepared to intervene. The cognitive state, (e.g., impairment of logic or other intellectual capabilities), thought process, and behaviors (such as motor activity and disruption of speech patterns) are the symptom categories observed, documented, and classified.

Hypomania

The first stage of mania might be called the *hypomanic period*. The mood is predominantly euphoric. The cognitive state is characterized by expansiveness of thought, grandiose ideas, and over-confidence. Thought process is coherent with a tendency to ramble. Behaviors noted include a beginning of pressured speech, some hypermotor activity, and an excessive display of humor. Frequent compliments to others and requests that at first seem logical and rational are also seen. A patient in this phase is friendly, happy, verbal and outgoing, the "social butterfly" of the unit.

Stage Two

The second stage is marked by an increased intensity of behaviors, greater disorganized cognition, and disrupted thought processes. Many patients spend money freely and may incur serious debt. The mood is generally irritable. The classic symptoms appear: frequent changing of clothes and wearing bizarre or multiple outfits at one time. The grandiose thinking takes on a paranoid flavor. Delusions become apparent, usually centering on religious or political ideation. Grandiosity of delusions is common, such as beliefs that the patient has important connections to religious or political people. Sleep patterns are interrupted. Staff will note patients sleeping a mere 2–3 hours per 24-hour period, and often sleeping at irregular, inappropriate times.

Stage Three

The intensity of stage 3 is striking; it is not seen, however, in every manic patient. Whereas the stage-2 patient's delusions and paranoia make interventions difficult, the stage-3 patient can rarely respond to verbal intervention of staff. Other major characteristics of stage 3 include: hallucinations, disorientation to time, place, or person, and severe panic (patients will often report that they feel their head is going to "explode"). The patient responds to all stimuli in the environment, even when it has no relation to the patient. The patient is physiologically exhausted, yet rarely sleeps.

The significance of recognizing the progressive stages of manic illness for the nurse is the ability to intervene successfully for the needs of the patient. (For more details, see intervention, p. 188. Frequently, the nurse can be "caught up" in the charisma of the early phase, only to find her- or himself unprepared for the more severe manifestations of stages 2 and 3. Thus, the nurse is using energy to struggle with his or her own lost objectivity rather than the patient's need for help. As a result of the nurse's slowness to respond, the patient, and often the entire milieu, can be disrupted before the staff begins to take action. At this point, intervention is much more complex and difficult.

INTERACTIONAL ENIGMAS

Along with identification of individual characteristics of the manic patient, the nurse in the milieu must also be aware of the classic interaction patterns of the manic. These patterns are not just problems of coping for the manic, but represent real destructive potential to the therapeutic milieu, and result in constant relationship failure for not only the manic person, but the other patients with whom he or she is involved. Janowsky et al. (1970) has delineated the "interpersonal maneuvers" seen in mania that create havoc for the patient and those around him/her.

The nurse may experience the manic as uncannily able to shift responsibility for his/her actions onto others. This projection is subtle, and frequently others involved are not aware that they have suddenly accepted the burden of the manic's rationalizations for a wide variety of questionable behavior or thoughts. A typical response would include a quite convincing list of other's foibles that have made it impossible for the manic to cooperate with a particular milieu norm, such as meal times.

Others' self-esteem is a target of manic interchanges. Because the manic experiences him or herself as able to control vast numbers of others, she or he readily uses attacks on other's self esteem (or conversely, building up other's self esteem) to control relationships. A typical interaction may begin with the manic praising aspects of the nurse's work, followed by a demand for some special favor or extra attention. If the nurse responds to the manic's demands, the nurse receives positive feedback. If not, his or her vulnerabilities are quickly discovered and attacked.

Frequently, this is a subtle process. The nurse becomes entangled in the manic patient's flattery, and may even verbally denegrate themselves or confess a weakness in response to their embarrassment due to the flattery. This material is then used by the manic in a successful ego attack after the patient has escalated and the nurse tries to limit some of the behavior. As a result, this false relationship built on pseudo-compliments, is doomed to failure. The nurse feels betrayed, helpless, and angry. The manic has once again found a foil for his or her engaging, yet pathological, patterns of interacting.

The nurse interacting with the manic patient may find these power struggle exchanges increasingly frustrating. Such struggles can begin as early as the admission process. Each demand by the patient seems to be a simple request, when the nurse focuses only on the request and not the whole pattern of the interaction, but the nurse can become enmeshed in this process—until the manic is out-of-bounds. When the nurse refuses cooperation, the manic targets in on the nurse for his or her rigidity and lack of fairness. Such complaints about one nurse are then used by the patient to elicit the cooperation of another "more equitable" staff member to gain the concession. The patient will continue to test and challenge in this manner, often drawing others into the interactions.

These dysfunctional interaction cycles interfere with the patient's ability to relate to others or to gain healthy rewards from a therapeutic relationship. The nurse who is able to identify such cycles when they occur, is prepared to intervene therapeutically by interrupting such dysfunction communication. Thus, there is greater ability to prevent enmeshment in the patient's skewed worldview, and greater potential for successful intervention towards the patient's well-being.

Case Example

Marty, a 32-year-old lawyer, was admitted to the unit through the emergency room. His loud, pressured speech was immediately apparent to all as he came down the hall, greeting everyone in his path and stopping frequently to look into various rooms. Each object he spied would introduce a new topic to his sentences. To one patient, he introduced himself as the mayor of a nearby town. As he spoke to others, he was quick to compliment them on their dress or hair. It was learned that he had recently purchased two automobiles and had not slept for over 72 hours. Marty's explaination of his hospitalization was that his boss "forced" him into it out of jealousy for Marty's great success in his career.

MILIEU

The milieu of a psychiatric unit is comprised of the physical space, patients, physicians, nurses, and other personnel. Another important component is the norms and values—spoken and unspoken—that guide the interactions, activities, and treatments. Each milieu is unique. A therapeutic milieu is one in which all components interact successfully to help persons develop effective communication, socially acceptable coping styles, and insight into behavior patterns. The theme of a milieu may then be defined according to the philosophy and function of its component parts.

Different types of milieu exist, e.g., a milieu that uses a token system can be characterized as highly structured, and specifically goal-oriented. One that emphasizes social interaction is considered less structured and may emphasize democratic processes as well.

The physical arrangement of a hospital unit influences the tone of the milieu. Tone refers to patient-activity level, anxiety level, neediness, or any significant event that effects the patient population. The physical plant that is large, and broken-up into nooks and crannies can obstruct observation of patient activities. The staff may then play more of a policing role in order to provide protection for patients. If a unit has private rooms, a boisterous patient can be isolated in order to decrease stimulation for that patient and others. Public areas that are roomy and well-furnished may enhance performance of appropriate behavior by creating a home-like versus institutional atmosphere.

While more planning has gone into modern psychiatric units, many treatment settings are renovated medical or surgical floors. On such units, staff's creativity in the use of space to encourage socially acceptable interactions can be challenged. Even with an "ideal" physical plant, a patient experiencing a manic episode can raise the anxiety level of the entire patient population if the components comprising the milieu are not therapeutically mobilized.

Mobilizing a milieu to set limits on the manic patient's behavior, while helping other patients to understand and tolerate the illness, is dependent on staff's ability to communicate with each other, particularly when patient needs are high. The nurse working with the manic patient must clearly convey to the patient's peers which specific behaviors are appropriate, which are not, and consequences attached to those inappropriate behaviors. All staff must especially involve themselves with monitoring the manic patient's behavior and other patients' reactions to it. Consistent communication of this information will help decrease the manic patient's effect on the milieu because staff who are involved with the other patients can successfully guide them away from the engaging appeal of the manic. Finally, visibility of staff on the unit is another key aspect of milieu. If no staff are out on the unit to observe destructive interactions, no intervention will occur.

In summary, a therapeutic milieu is comprised of the interaction of patients and staff on a unit. Key variables to be consistently aware of are monitoring of the physical plant, clear communication among staff (and patients with staff), consistent limit-setting, and a sharing of intervention strategies with each other to get support. These variables effect the success of treatment modalities and philosophy of every individual unit. The following case example illustrates the sensitivity of a manic patient to a specific milieu.

Case Example

Although cooperative with the admission procedure, Marty is ambivalent about hospitalization. His "charming" demeanor quickly changes to irritability when questions are raised regarding his symptoms or illness. Demonstrating his denial, he frequently changes the subject by complimenting staff on their appearance and manner. He becomes sexually provocative with these remarks, engaging staff in dealing with this behavior and their own embarrassment rather than placing limits on his behaviors and focusing on the real issues of the interview.

As the interview continues, Marty often interjects questions about the hospital, rules, food, and activities on the unit. Apologies preface each interruption, yet they continue. He expresses praise and gratitude when the nurse responds to his questions. It seems impossible to refocus him.

Later, on the unit, his first stop is the snack kitchen where he meets two adolescent patients discussing their anger about being in the hospital. Marty tells them that they certainly seem to be normal and encourages them to sign out of the hospital or just leave. He stresses that he is a lawyer, impressing the adolescents, and intensifying their desire to leave the hospital. So they begin to plot an escape. After the brief encounter in the kitchen, Marty slips into the day area where a group of borderline patients are discussing the effectiveness of their physicians in helping them to get better. He quickly becomes part of the group by introducing himself as a lawyer and proceeds to lecture on consumer rights. A nurse approaches him to take a tranquilizer ordered by the physician. Marty refuses the medication, eliciting the group's help in assuring the nurse that he is under control and managing well on the unit. The nurse, feeling outnumbered, agrees to hold the medication, but indicates that he should take a time-out in his room. She charts the medication as refused and documents that the patient is able to response to verbal limits. Marty stays in his room for 5 minutes.

In a matter of hours, Marty has met everyone on the unit and has presented himself as a patient advocate, vitally interested in helping all overcome the "oppressive" nature of unit procedures. Communication between staff and patients breaks down to polarity. Throughout these events, Marty maintains his neutrality, successfully avoiding taking any responsibility for generating these interactions.

Three days later, Marty's grandiose presentation of self begins to wear thin. Other patients begin complaining that Marty constantly interrupts and goes in and out of their rooms. Some staff have noticed that shift reports and other discussions about Marty almost always end in staff arguments about whether Marty is "out of control or not." Those that do place limits on Marty's behavior are attacked as unfair. Marty frequently responds to these limits by demanding to be discharged.

Case Analysis

Marty's case exemplifies common characteristics of hypomanic behavior (see previous classification, p. 183). He begins, at admission, to exhibit the enhanced perceptiveness that leads to rapid, nonmutual, intense relationships. Quickly launching into control issues, he uses flattery, provocative behavior, and intimidation to manipulate others. By using such unconscious ploys, he denies his illness and avoids responsibility for behavior or for cooperating with treatment.

Staff members were slow to intervene, a major danger in the treatment of mania. This occurs because staff get caught up in the "charisma" of the patient and fail to establish prompt boundaries, or limits, on his behavior. Thus, the patient's behavior has escalated before interventions begin.

For instance, the nurse in the admission interview became embarrassed and ineffective. A better response is to acknowledge his or her feelings, set a limit on the behavior, restate the purpose of the interview, and refocus on the topic.

Acknowledge, Restate, and Refocus

When the nurse acknowledges his or her feelings, the flattery ploy of the patient fails, helping the patient reconnect with the topic at hand. This also provides boundaries for the patient, as the nurse states the feeling and that the manic's behavior is inappropriate to the setting. Such verbal skills must be utilized numerous times with the patient in every interaction. Patient response to this consistency may be more agitation, but usually the patient will become more calm and cooperative.

Day Room Interaction

The nurse was unsuccessful in medicating Marty because he was given free-roam of the unit. It is usually much more helpful to keep the patient in his room, where interactions can be private and over-stimulation avoided. In this setting, Marty would have been more likely to cooperate with the nurse. Although confinement to room may not be indicated in every case, in patients with extreme behavior such as Marty's, it can be a major step in establishing a working relationship early in the hospitalization.

Limit Access to Milieu, Medicate

Limited access proves valuable in focusing the patient and prevents en-trapments that would then have to be repaired or would escalate the patient.

As seen in the case example, behavior that is not responded-to or controlled, can escalate not only the patient's behavior, but disrupt the entire milieu. This happens, whether the behavior is hypomanic, such as in Marty's case, or an active episode of mania. Nursing intervention must focus on both corrective individual responses for the patient, and constant monitoring and intervention at the community level.

STRATEGIES FOR NURSING INTERVENTION

The major focus of nursing intervention in the treatment of both acute and chronic episodes of mania, must remain on the actual issues of the illness, rather than specific content in which the patient may invest; e.g., the intervention focus is the patients' lack of judgment, secondary to the illness, and not the fact that patients feel they have a right to give all their clothes to their roommates. Or, the focus is poor impulse control, secondary to the illness, not whether patients feel it is important to interrupt others.

By continuing to focus on the treatment issues of the illness, the nurse can provide patient education, avoid power struggles, and bring the patient to an understanding of the denial process that is so active in mania.

Due to patients' hypersensitivities to stimulation, as well as their distractibility, it is preferable to have most nurse–patient interactions in a private setting. In the acute phase, manic patients may already be confined to their rooms; as medication begins to help, however, and patients move more freely in the milieu, opportunities for private discussion of patients' behavior and treatment must be directed by the nurse. Limit-setting and discussion of patients' issues are best done in such a setting to prevent patients' bringing into the discussion all others in the immediate area. Thus, both patients and the milieu are protected from escalation and disruption.

In a situation where patients have appealed to others in a discussion involving their behavior, the first intervention is to stop the patient and refocus to a private setting. When this fails, patients are able to elicit others in evaluating the "fairness" or "logic" of theirs and the nurse's behavior, rather than the manic symptoms that are in need of control. The nurse can best manage the content by bringing patients back to the fact that this is a problem in the illness. The nurse may also state that other patients can be most helpful to manic patients by not allowing themselves to continue the interaction. The nurse must keep in mind the original goal of providing privacy and confidentiality, even when patients do not have the judgment to seek this.

PATIENT EDUCATION

Manic-depressive illness is a chronic disease for many patients. A key factor in controlling the illness and its effect on the patient and family is patient/family education. Patients with bipolar illness, similar to those with other chronic diseases, experience a wide variety of responses, from denial, to anger, to acceptance. With mania, the denial often becomes a major block to treatment and education efforts. Hence the need is for the nurse to carefully assess patient progress and readiness to learn before moving into active work for patient/family education. The objective is to replace the dysfunctional responses to the illness with informed goal-directed behavior to control and alleviate the destructive potential of this chronic disease on the patient's life.

Preparing the patient and family to manage a bipolar illness starts with the understanding that this disease is chronic and it is not always under the patient's control. Frequently, it is necessary to allay the families' guilt, that it is someone's "fault" the illness occurred. This goal is extremely difficult to achieve and may only be started while the patient is hospitalized.

Another important educational goal entails familiarizing the patient, family, and other staff regarding interventions utilized in treatment. All must realize the importance of gradual entry into the milieu, close observation, and steady progression into control of the behaviors with medication. The patient often attempts to thwart these efforts, for it is common in the illness for the patient to be noncompliant with the treatment regime. When other patients and staff accept the manic's ploys as caused by an illness, the patient's treatment can proceed in a timely and least disruptive manner.

Education should begin immediately when a patient in an acute manic state is admitted to the unit. The responses of the staff and fellow patients to the manic's disruptiveness, constant interruptions, and charm and wit, should consistently contain two major points: the behavior is due to the illness, and nursing treatment will monitor the safety of both the patient, and others, plus active management of the presenting behavior. Other patients especially need to hear that the manic patient's response to treatment (i.e., medications, seclusion, primary therapy) will take time. Thus, the nurse can successfully deal with the individual patient while maintaining a focus on the therapeutic needs of the total milieu. The manic patient needs to consistently hear that disruptive behaviors are caused by the illness and treatment is aimed to prevent embarrassment and help the individual learn about the illness and its impact on the patient and others.

Thus, each milieu-intervention strategy is accompanied by the opportunity for both the patient and others to become educated about the illness. To either intervene without education or try education without the intervention eventually leads to frustration of the overall goals: managing the behavior, the mileu's response to that behavior, and preparing the patient for life-long coping with the illness.

MEDICATIONS

Central to managing the patient's behavior is the nurse's thoughtful utilization of the prescribed medication regimen, both routine and p.r.n. In collaboration with the physician, the nurse uses judgment and close observation to monitor changes in the patient's behavior. This requires thorough knowledge of the patient's premorbid functioning. This is crucial when discussing changes in route, dosage, or frequency. The nurse's observations are a key factor in early detection of side effects, which must be of particular importance in rapid tranquilization of acute manic states. Physician–nurse dialogue is vital for consistency of effort and ensures a clear message to the patient concerning medications. In the experience of these authors, medications are used most commonly to obtain 2 major outcomes: controlling the symptoms of an acute manic episode, and remission of the chemical imbalance that has caused the manic episode.

In most cases, both of these outcomes must be worked on simultaneously in the hospitalization. Since control of the symptoms usually occurs more rapidly than remission, patients will commonly receive a major tranquilizer such as Haldol, Mellaril, Prolixin, etc., while Lithium Carbonate or Tegretol therapy is building to a therapeutic dose.

It is in the area of p.r.n. medication that the nurse must be the most informed and knowledgeable. Resources on pharmacology, extrapyramidal syndromes, and rapid tranquilization should be utilized consistently to prepare the nurse to function successfully with p.r.n.s for the manic patient. The nurse's judgment and documentation of behavior changes, especially as they may correlate with blood levels of the medications, is vital. Many nurses are chronic "under-utilizers" of p.r.n. medication for mania usually because of an inadequate premorbid assessment. This exposes both patients and milieu to disruption and interpersonal pain that is totally unnecessary. Constant observation of patients' moods, thought processes, and motor activities must be made and correlated with adequate administration of p.r.n. medications.

Finally, opportunity for patients' education concerning medications must be consistently utilized. As the nurse becomes more informed, she or he can be a major resource to patients' education about medications and what to expect from them, as well as learning to be compliant with the medication regimen.

STRUCTURE

The last component of milieu management of mania involves structuring the milieu to ameliorate the presenting symptomatology of the manic patient as well as reactions in the milieu. This is especially important to nurses when their judgments about manic patients' mobility, visibility, and input into milieu issues have to prevail over the manic patients' desire for compulsive interaction—or over others in the milieu becoming involved in the unhealthy interaction.

As each milieu is different, the specific structures that can be utilized will vary. The authors have found the following helpful:

1. Structuring specific consequences for problem behavior, e.g., loud and interrupting behavior results in the patient being restricted to his or her room for a specific period.
2. Consequences for inappropriate behaviors, as well as structured activity, should be simple and easily communicated to the patient and others— especially across shifts—for consistency.
3. The care plan can be an effective tool for clearly identifying behavioral outcomes. The plan should articulate:
    *   The patient's daily schedule, which should be very regimented at first with controls on interacting time. As the patient improves, more flexibility is possible. It is important to be specific about where the patient may go on the unit. The schedule should include exercise and quiet time.

- Intervention strategies that are useful when the patient does not respond to verbal limits. This may include progressive steps from escorting the patient to his or her room, or may include a quiet room or restraints if necessary.
- It is usually recommended that a manic patient not be treated in group therapy.* If this treatment is ordered, it should be noted specifically which meetings are excluded and if others, such as community meetings, may be included.
- As the patient improves, the care plan can include negotiated behavioral cues that can be used by staff to unobtrusively signal the patient when he or she is escalating. This is one more step in the patient's regaining self-esteem and control over his or her own behavior.

4. The patient's sleep pattern should be monitored and recorded. Structured sleep time can then be planned to accomodate the patient's individuality, yet move toward healthier sleep-cycle establishment (See Chapter 5 on sleep patterns).
5. Utilize the community meeting to further enhance patient education regarding mania, providing a forum for patients to talk about their feelings and reactions to the manic patient; reaffirming safety on the unit, and mobilizing the milieu from a reactive stance to helpful interactions with the manic patient.

Regular interdisciplinary treatment planning can be helpful in outlining other milieu structures that may be added to or removed from the patient's treatment as needed. This might include, occupational therapy projects, participation in off-unit activities, joining the milieu for meals, extended visiting hours, etc.

Finally, in considering structure, the nurse must keep in mind the continuous intra-nursing and interdisciplinary collaboration that must occur for success to be achieved. This collaboration, with careful timing of interventions based on the patient's behavior, will bring the best hope for meshing treatment needs of the individual with the needs of the milieu.

REFERENCES

Carlson, G. A., & Goodwin, F. K. (1973). The stages of mania: A longitudinal analysis of the manic episode. *Archives of General Psychiatry, 28,* 221–228.
Diagnostic and Statistical Manual of Mental Disorders. 3rd Edition. (1980). Washington, D.C. American Psychiatric Association. 206–210.

*The authors recommend that a staff member be seated next to the manic patient in any group the patient may attend. This helps the patient maintain control and facilitates escorting the patient out of the group should it be necessary.

Janowsky, D. S., Leff, M., & Epstein, R. S. (1970). Playing the manic game: Interpersonal maneuvers of the acutely manic patient. *Archives of General Psychiatry, 22,* 252–261.

ANNOTATED BIBLIOGRAPHY

Belmaker, R. H., Pragg van H. M. (1980). *Mania, an evolving concept.* Spectrum Publications Inc. Jamaica, N.Y.
   Perhaps the most inclusive book found on mania, Belmaker and Pragg, covers the concept from many perspectives. The subjective experience of mania, psychosocial precipitants, management, and the hypomanic personality in history are chapters applicable to this chapter. The remainder of the book looks at the differentiation between acute mania and schizophrenia.

Dixon, D. L. (1981). *Manic depression: An overview.* Journal of Psychiatric Nursing and Mental Health Services 19:28–31.
   This article provides theories of mania. The predominant theories discussed are the psychoanalytical and physiological. Lithium therapy and nursing implications are highlighted. Correlations are made between lithium tolerance and behavioral symptoms. One correlation that is not found in nursing journals is the patient's high tolerance to lithium during mania and low tolerance when the patient is stabilized.

Haber, J., et al (1979). *Comprehensive psychiatric nursing: The client who threatens self concept.* New York: McGraw Hill.
   A framework for assessment and intervention with the manic patient is discussed. Mania is divided into three stages. Interventions focus on the patient who is manic and are appropriate for undergraduate nursing students. The chapter does not discuss the effects of mania on an inpatient unit or the ways in which the staff can create a milieu to effectively treat the chaos which may arise.

Moos, R. H. (1974). *Evaluating treatment environments: A sociological approach: The effects of treatment milieus.* New York: John Wiley & Sons, 331–335.
   Variables of a nursing unit are identified. Size of the physical plant, staffing patterns, staff morale, and unit philosophy are emphasized as variables that effect treatment outcomes. While the article does not address mania, it does provide a framework for mobilizing concrete variables to create a milieu effective in the treatment of the manic patient.

11

Depressed Elderly in the Inpatient Psychiatric Milieu

Susan Anderson
Debra Sivesind

Affective disorders do not discriminate in favor of age; in fact, the elderly are probably more vulnerable than any other age group to their onslaught. Explanations for this increased incidence come from biological and sociological, as well as psychological frameworks. The range of affective disorders in the elderly is comparable to that of younger patients. The manifestations and interventions, however, may vary considerably.

Elderly patients are frequently hospitalized. The elderly patient may gain entry to the inpatient setting because his or her clinical picture is not clearly determined. An affective disorder may be only one of a series of possible explanations for the individual's symptomatology. Weight loss, changes in cognitive function, apathy, and complaints of somatic distress are commonly present in illness states other than affective disorders. In fact, an affective disorder may represent the final diagnostic option considered for the patient. Even when an affective disorder is diagnosed for the elderly patient, the decreased physiological status or the presence of concurrent medical problems may necessitate inpatient hospitalization for treatment. Psychiatric nurses in an inpatient milieu will become increasingly involved with such patients.

Psychiatric nurses are in a key position to assess and intervene with the hospitalized elderly person experiencing an affective disorder. Nursing's concept

NURSING INTERVENTIONS IN DEPRESSION   Copyright © 1985 by Grune & Stratton, Inc.
ISBN 0-8089-1710-2   All rights of reproduction in any form reserved.

of the holistic person allows the nurse to grasp accurately the complex nature of assessment and intervention required. Elderly patients are notoriously unable to identify the source of their distress. Nursing assessment can, therefore, incorporate direct observation of the patient over a 24-hour period in addition to the individual's self report. The nurse's assessment combines sound understanding of normal aging and the pathology of an affective disorder, as well as recognition of the impact of physiological alterations on milieu participation.

The purpose of this chapter is to discuss elements of nursing assessment and intervention relevant to the nurse clinician practicing with an inpatient population that includes elderly patients experiencing an affective disorder.

ASSESSMENT

As stated earlier, elderly patients do not manifest their affective disorders in the more straightforward fashion of younger patients. They can rarely identify an affective disorder as a source of distress. In addition, their longevity may place them at risk due to their physiological fragility and concurrent medical problems. They may be socially vulnerable as well, due to relocation or loss of friends and family.

Each facet in the clinical picture of the elderly patient contains vital information for formulation and implementation of nursing care. Nursing assessment must be comprehensive in scope, including information collected in an initial interview with the patient and information gained over time. A mental status exam, a historical picture of the patient including his perception of events leading up to hospitalization, a social and family assessment, perhaps a work history, and a functional physical assessment including a drug history are usually initially included. Other elements of the assessment are better deferred, e.g., the patient's functioning in the milieu is often a better indication than a mental status exam of the degree of actual impairment the patient experiences as a result of cognitive dysfunction (Ebersole & Hess, 1981). Additional diagnostic testing is frequently helpful in determining the nature of the patient's difficulty.

Mental Status Exam

Upon introducing herself to the patient, the nurse may begin to assess elements of the mental status exam. Actually, the exam can proceed throughout the initial nurse–patient interaction without much demand placed on the patient. Although the content organization of the mental-status exam can vary, the elements themselves are fairly consistent. For purposes of this discussion, the elements are organized as:

1. Appearance and behavior.
2. Affect and mood.
3. Thought content.
4. Thought processes.
5. Perceptual experience (Johnson et al., 1975).

Appearance and Behavior

In assessing the patient's appearance and behavior the nurse observes dress and grooming, posture, facial expression, eye contact, speech, level of motor behavior, and unusual mannerisms. When dress and grooming are appropriate rather than bizarre, observation yields clues regarding the patient's perception of him- or herself as an older adult. Stylish dress makes a different statement than does a grandmotherly (or grandfatherly) approach to adorning oneself. When dress and grooming are disheveled or bizarre, they are of diagnostic importance. Disheveled dress, even slight in degree, may be an early indication of chronic organic brain syndrome. Bizarre, provocative dress may indicate a bipolar disorder in a manic phase or a more histrionic character style. The examiner begins to formulate some tentative hypotheses regarding the meaning of each piece of data and looks to other areas of assessment for confirmation. No one item can stand alone diagnostically; the entire picture is of crucial importance.

Slumped posture, sad facial expression, slowed speech and motor behavior, and limited eye contact all contribute to a clinical presentation of depression. In the elderly, however, the facial expression of a depressed patient may be extremely apathetic and flat. The nurse may describe a facial expression as "bewildered" or "frightened" and motor activity as "increased." The signs may reflect situational or chronic anxiety, or anxiety associated with an awareness of decreased cognitive function made even more obvious by the novel situation of hospital admission. Hypomanic elderly patients rarely display the characteristic hyperactive, hyperverbal behavior of younger patients with this disorder. The difference may be due to a general decrease in activity that often accompanies aging. It is usually more helpful to rely on historical data for the diagnosis of a bipolar disorder rather than to search for the characteristic symptomatology found in younger patients.

Affect and Mood

Changes in affect and mood are considered a cardinal sign in depression. Elderly patients experiencing a depressive affective disorder often display the characteristic mood of fixed sadness. Concurrent medical illness or pain, however, can mask the significant affect. A classic example is Parkinson's Disease. The nurse may find that she or he needs to rely on other elements of the assessment to confirm the diagnostic impression. A diagnosis of Parkinson's does not necessarily rule out the concurrent psychiatric intervention. The medical diagnosis merely makes the affective diagnosis more difficult.

An elderly patient can express a somatic symptom as the chief complaint. A significant expression of affect and mood is the degree of anxiety and distress displayed in relationship to the somatic symptom. When the level of distress is out of proportion to what one might normally expect from the particular symptomatology, a depressive equivalent is suspected. When the nurse recognizes this phenomenon in a patient, she needs to take note and inquire about the onset of the somatic source of distress. The nature of losses or other stressful events occurring in the patient's life around the same time as the onset of the disorder frequently give even more credence to the impression of depressive equivalent.

The euphoric mood of hypomania appears in many elderly patients with this disorder. Others, however, demonstrate the irritability and lability also common in bipolar patients. Examination of other portions of the assessment, particularly as to whether the patient has previously experienced mood swings, can be helpful to the nurse in formulating a clinical impression.

Thought Content

The area of thought content can present problems in objective assessment when the normal content for the elderly patient seems depressing to the nurse doing the assessment. Normal portions of thought content for the elderly include a review of the individual's life with some increased focus on past over present or future events (Butler, 1963; Burnside, 1981). In contrast to younger patients, the diagnostic significance of these findings is decreased with the elderly. In assessing thought content, the nurse listens for the meaning attached to content as well as the content itself. The nurse may ask if relatively unimportant events are construed with more significant meaning, or if the meaning is construed in such a way that perfectly human shortcomings become catastrophic character flaws. The nurse may question if there is a preoccupation with such events without evidence of psychological movement or working through. These findings are more indicative of an affective disorder. Yet, thought content reflecting some past-tense orientation, particularly with evidence of a realistic and constructive working-through of events, can be interpreted as part of the normal development of the aging individual.

Practitioners sometimes experience difficulty in differentiating grief and depression. Historically, length of time required to resolve the loss was used as a relevant criteria. This is no longer the case. Currently, a pattern of less intensely felt dysphoria over time is considered a key distinguishing factor in grief although particular events that remind the patient of the loss may heighten the dysphoric mood temporarily (Simos, 1979). When assessing an elderly patient with dysphoric mood, the nurse should seek some history of onset and intensity of the mood and the relationship of the intensity to other events, such as anniversaries.

Assessing for vegetative signs of depression is another useful measure for differentiating grief and depression when mental status findings indicate dysphoric mood. Presence of vegetative signs is positive indication for chemotherapeutic intervention in addition to relationship work (Corbett, 1980). Simos (1979) offers a series of questions about the nature of the patient's expressed dysphoria that may also be helpful in differentiation. She also points out the need to consider whether personality characteristics of the patient make a realistic working-through of grief difficult.

Delusional thought content occurs in the elderly with affective disorders as well as those with more clear-cut psychoses. Depressive delusions are somatically focused, often describing in vivid detail the death and decay the patient imagines is occurring within his or her own body. A delusion reflecting depression can also assume the form of an idea of reference: that a horribly unfortunate event affecting many people has been precipitated in some way by an act of the depressed individual. Gradiose delusions and preoccupations of a sexual nature in the elderly can indicate a diagnosis of bipolar depression, manic phase. However, the nurse must rule out the possibility that verbal or behavioral expression of sexual thought content could be related to an organic process loosening inhibitions before assuming that an affective disorder exists.

The nurse must be aware of any sign of suicidal ideation to thought content in the mental-status exam. As a group, the elderly have a high rate of successful suicide. The content may be passively expressed as a wish or desire. When the nurse identifies such content, he or she needs to include an assessment of the risk factors present for a successful attempt. She must also identify any indirect self-destructive behaviors the patient utilizes since there is some evidence that one can substitute for the other (Nelson & Farberow, 1976).

Thought Processes

Thought processes in the elderly may be influenced by an affective disorder, cognitive disorder, or some combination of the two. The differentiation of dementia from the pseudodementia of depression is problematic, requiring skill as well as thoroughness in assessment.

Thought processes can be divided into the subelements of orientation, memory, intellect, thought-flow or stream, and judgment. Thought-flow is assessed contextually in the initial interview. Depressed elderly frequently demonstate a slowing of thought and thought blocking. It is important to distinguish this phenomena from the trailing off of an incomplete thought that may occur with an organic process. Increased speed of thought and flight of ideas, indicative of a manic phase in a bipolar disorder, are seen in the elderly, although degree of speed is decreased compared to that of a younger patient. Often, the interviewer finds it more helpful to attune to the form of the thought-flow rather than to its speed.

Whereas most of the previous portions of the entire exam can proceed

within the course of an admission interview, assessment of orientation and memory usually requires more specific activity on the part of the patient. The elderly
patient frequently experiences such demands as threatening, and the anxiety
provoked by the threat can negatively influence performance. Some authors
suggest a contextual exam to circumvent the threatening experience (Pfeiffer,
1975). However, others point out that a contextual exam can only be considered
a screening mechanism and that a more detailed exam is usually necessary for a
diagnostic differentiation of depression and chronic or acute organic brain syndrome (Smyer et al., 1979).

Based on the above discussion, the most satisfactory approach is to be
guided by cues gained in the interview thus far. If the patient gives a coherent
accounting of events leading up to hospitalization, accurately describes his or her
physical condition, special concerns, and progresses through admission paper-
work, including dates and signatures, the nurse can reasonably assume that
memory and orientation are adequate. If patient's participation in the milieu later
indicates that further assessment is necessary, a more thorough exam can be
completed.

Often, however, the admission interview indicates a fluctuating level of
consciousness, a short attention span, or other signs of potential difficulty in the
area of memory and orientation. Any such observations suggest the need for a
more thorough assessment than that which can be accomplished contextually.
Each nurse needs to develop a style of gathering this data that is comfortable to
her and is as comforting as possible for the patient. Introducing the topic directly
is often the easiest approach. In terms of timing, it is usually most helpful to wait
for a point in the interview when the patient has become accustomed to his or her
surroundings and to the nurse.

Orientation assessment consists of orientation to person, place, and time.
Time orientation should be elicited by asking the patient the day of the week,
date, year, and possibly time of day. The information is initially recorded as the
patient states it, without interpretation. However, the nurse should also note the
patient's response when he or she does not readily know the information; i.e., if
the patient admits to ignorance, fills in or confabulates, or becomes angry at the
question, such actions give a fairly clear indication of the patient's inability to
cope with cognitive changes (Wolanin & Phillips, 1981). When the patient is
unable to give the requested information, and this finding is noted, it is helpful to
offer cues from the environment and assess the patient's ability to utilize these.

Judgment is a discrete area of mental status. The patient's ability to utilize
adequate judgment, however, can help to compensate for decreased functioning
in the areas of orientation and recent memory. Ideally, judgment is assessed in
the milieu based on the conditions presented to the patient, e.g., what behavior
does the patient exhibit when confronted with hunger or thirst, and no food or
drink is readily available, and how adaptive are these behaviors? The nurse can

also interpret assessment of judgment from the description the patient offers of his or her living situation, illness, and the patient's response to it.

Memory is divided into categories of immediate recall, recent memory, and remote memory. Immediate recall can be assessed by telling the patient to remember a brief statement or short series of objects and then immediately asking the patient to repeat these items. If the patient is unable to speak, the same task might be accomplished using a series of objects available in the environment. The patient is asked to point them out to the nurse in the same order in which they were identified (Wolanin & Phillips, 1981).

Recent memory is often contextually assessed by requesting a description of events occurring around hospitalization. If these cannot be verified, it is preferable to allow several hours of milieu events to transpire and then to request the patient's accounting of these. Remote memory can likewise be examined as part of collecting a patient's history, provided that events can be verified by family or significant others. If this is not possible, it may be helpful to draw on the patient's memory of significant historical events (Wolanin & Phillips, 1981).

Regardless of the factual findings in a mental status exam, it is important to determine how many changes in cognitive function actually interfere with the patient's ability to manage common activities in everyday life (Ebersole & Hess, 1981). In order to make such determination, the assessments should be repeated, since the patient requires time to accustom him- or herself to the hospital environment. As the patient becomes accustomed, his or her performance may improve.

Perceptual Experience

The assessment of perceptual experience can be conveniently divided into two areas: perception as belief or insight, and perception as a sensory experience.

Very early in the initial assessment, the nurse needs to elicit the patient's perception regarding the precipitating events of hospitalization. Elderly patients vary tremendously in the way they attribute causes: some respond with somatic complaints or descriptions of physical illness, some may blame relatives or close friends for unnecessarily pushing the hospitalization, and others respond with a somewhat incomplete psychologically oriented answer. Regardless of the manner in which concern is expressed, the patient is providing important information regarding him- or herself as a person as well as how the patient views the affective experience. The nurse must actively and empathetically listen to not only the fashion in which the patient expresses him- or herself but also to the factual content of information in order to discern what the patient's subjective experience is.

When the elderly patient attributes the distress to losses and changes in his or her life in a relatively straightforward fashion, the assessment is easily completed. As with any patient, the nurse, by questioning, assists in expanding and elaborating on the patient's description. Frequently, however, the elderly patient responds with physical or somatic complaints rather than psychologically oriented answers.

As the nurse listens to the patient's recitation of physical concerns, he or she begins to sort out what this information means. The patient may be describing common physiological manifestations of depression, such as sleeplessness or a sense of increased fatigue, heightened pain sensitivity, loss of appetite, and constipation. Perhaps the picture is one of a depressive equivalent with a sense of unusual, otherwise unexplicable, pain or similar symptoms. When the nurse begins to sense that either might be the case, she or he gently tests the patient's perception by inquiring as to the original onset of symptoms and attempts to expand on events that were occurring in the patient's life at the same time. An important observation is whether the patient can begin to relate the physiological experience to the affective one. The patient's ability to do so is an important indication of potential for insight. Making such a connection also tends to reduce the demoralization that is usually a part of any psychiatric disorder, which is inherently reassuring to the patient (Frank, 1975). A patient who is unable to make such a mind–body connection can provide the nurse with at least a time frame for the onset of symptoms. As the interview proceeds and the nurse learns from the patient, family, or friends of other trauma experienced by the patient, he or she will want to keep in mind for potential correlation the time frame for the onset of the patient's physical symptoms. The information is helpful in confirming the nurse's hypothesis about the nature of the patient's symptoms even though the patient is not able to utilize the information at the time.

Sometimes patient complaints begin to describe a physical illness. The nurse needs to be familiar with common disease states that include depression or mood changes as part of their presenting picture. Most common in the elderly are endocrine dysfunction, metastatic disease, Parkinson's Disease, and mood changes related to drug treatment (Corbett, 1980).

The nurse needs to alert him- or herself to physical assessment findings likely in each of these disorders. This familiarity will allow the nurse to focus during the physical assessment. The nurse also needs to bear in mind that many chronic conditions are neither exclusively physical nor psychological. Some conditions may contain elements of *both* a treatable physical and psychological concern.

Occasionally, the patient expresses the affective disorder in a delusional fashion with sensory components associated. Examples of such expressions include the sense that one is rotting inside, that the patient's body is disintegrating, or the bowel is blocked. One very depressed patient told his nurse repeatedly that he smelled so awful that no one would want to be near him—an indirect expression of the delusional decay he felt secondary to his depression. Although a patient this depressed probably needs other measures, such as chemotherapy or electroshock therapy (ECT) before the impact of relationship work can be felt, it may still be helpful to briefly delve into the onset of the patient's concern in a way that is comforting to the patient and to attempt to make some correlation to his or her affective experience. It is also important to provide feedback to the patient that he or she is acceptable to you, the nurse, even though the patient may feel badly about him- or herself at this point. This type of delusional experience should be distinguished from hallucinations not so tied to the patient's affective experience. The presence of hallucinations may be indicative of a psychosis or a psychotic affective disorder. The other common sensory distortion is an illusion in which the patient misinterprets an actual sensory experience; e.g., one elderly patient noted to her nurse that she saw a snake on the floor instead of the telephone cord actually present. This phenomena is usually indicative of an organic process, and the patient in this example was later diagnosed to have a brain metastatic process.

Historical Picture

Obtaining a historical picture of the patient's distress is important. Core personality characteristics are fairly stable throughout adult life. Unless tied to some significant situational components, the onset of a marked personality change in late life is unusual, generally suggesting an organic rather than affective disorder (Corbett, 1980).

The information collected in a historical picture can include when the patient first began to feel differently, what was occurring in his or her life at that time, exactly how the patient perceives the changes experienced, and what the course of the distress has been from the time the patient first experienced it to the present. When the patient isolates distress in what seems to be a depressive equivalent, a delusional experience, or other aberration, it is helpful to refrain from challenging this experience until some of the surrounding data can be obtained. To challenge the patient prematurely may raise defenses and negatively impact the validity of any further information. After the nurse has inquired as to onset, other concurrent life events, and course, he or she can then usually test the patient's interpretation of experience.

Sometimes a patient expresses euphoria rather than distress, and anxiety and worry will be expressed by relatives rather than the patient. The nurse can ask the patient what his or her current experience is, how long the patient has felt this way, and whether this experience has ever occurred before. In determining if the experience is a bipolar disorder, it is important to ask about cyclical swings; if the patient ever feels that thoughts are moving much faster than usual, or that she or he needs far less rest than usual. A nurse can also question if the reverse is ever true. If the patient is unable to give an accurate historical account, some information may be obtained from secondary sources, such as family or friends.

The nurse may encounter a patient who is so immobilized by an affective disorder that he or she is nonverbal. The nonverbal patient demands special interview considerations. Nonverbal is different than nonresponsive. The nonresponsive patient demands rapid determination of level of consciousness and physical findings to identify the problem and appropriate intervention. The nonverbal patient may fluctuate in attention and nonverbal response to the interviewer but does not answer questions directly asked. When interviewing the patient, the nurse should first attempt to address the patient directly and establish eye contact, speaking slowly and clearly in a low tone of voice. The nurse should ask only yes, no, or very short-answer questions. Plenty of time should be allowed for reply as well as verbal interpretation of the patient's nonverbal responses to questions. If the patient is still not responding, the nurse might explain that she or he is going to ask the same question of the family or significant others but is hopeful that the patient will respond as well. The nurse needs to refer back to the patient throughout the interview and to continue to interpret the patient's nonverbal behavior.

Social and Family Assessment

Family or significant others are usually involved early in the patient's admission process. While the nurse establishes contact with the patient, as described earlier with a nonverbal patient, she or he also assesses the family and allies them in the treatment plan. The link between the presence and quality of support systems and the patient's well-being is not always clear. Sometimes the finding is that the patient's needs clearly outstretch support available, and the family—as well as the patient—become the focus of intervention in locating and working through appropriate placement. In assessment, the nurse will want to identify who is involved with the patient and what the quality of the relationship, familial or otherwise, is to that patient. It is important to identify all types of involvement, including long distance, financial, and telephone contacts. Overall number in the support system is important. Any recent losses within the support system must also be identified. Sometimes many individuals within the family system are grieving or depressed and are unable to be of assistance to the patient. Length of time involved with the patient is an important variable to be noted. The nurse may interview a patient involved in a late-life marriage or second marriage that took place recently while the individual was active and healthy. Sometimes a great deal of resentment or guilt exists in such a relationship when the patient becomes incapacitated with an affective disorder or a physical illness.

In addition to the preceding information the nurse will want to make a systems assessment of the family based on interaction with them in the interview. The nurse assesses if they are relatively open or if it is difficult to gain information. It is important to note whether anyone in the family functions as gatekeeper or decision-maker, and how decisions are reached. Usually the interview provides ample opportunity to observe decision-making processes. First-hand observation is generally more accurate than anything individuals can tell the nurse about what happens in their family. Keep in mind, however, that absent, long-distance members can maintain considerable control or influence. Do not discount this in the absence of their physical presence. Sometimes the process is such that the family system cannot reach any decision without a telephone conversation with another family member.

An awareness of historical dynamics that exist in most families, which may include sibling rivalry and mechanisms of esteem development, is important. The nurse will want to observe whether these tensions are still played out and to what degree they influence family interaction presently. In addition, the nurse needs to be aware of more pathological features of family interaction, such as scapegoating, labeling, or pseudomutuality, that may be present. Although in-depth family treatment is rarely the goal of an acute hospitalization, family system functioning can have dramatic impact on progress in basic treatment and disposition decisions. Elements of family system function must be identified and accomodated if short-term intervention is truly to remain short-term and effective.

The nurse may interview a patient with few or no real significant others. In this case it is important to identify whether a lifelong pattern exists or whether the situation is due to losses of meaningful relationships. Both findings have important implications. When it appears that the patient has characteristically maintained little or superficial involvement with others, the patient may be suffering from an affective disorder with underlying schizoid personality features. Such a finding influences the manner in which the nurse identifies goals for the patient within the milieu. No dramatic change in social functioning will be obtained by forcing interaction on such a patient.

When losses have created a void in the patient's number of relationships, implications for assessment include examining the patient's ability to grieve for the losses he or she has experienced. A second assessment is the identification of depletion anxiety (Verwoerdt, 1981). The patient may be quite anxious as she or he experiences resources falling away and is unable to find people to meet his or her needs. A social history that indicates frequent relocation can be a significant finding in an affective disorder. The patient may move often because unpleasant feelings are externalized to the environment again and again (Corbett, 1980).

Work History

Work history is closely related to social and family history. For many people, work has formed a central portion of their self-esteem and has been significant in their relationships with others. Examination of the patient's work experiences yields a more complete history of that patient's strengths. In addition, the nurse will want to be aware of how the process of retirement has taken place. Premature retirement, often related to physical concerns or fatigue, is a significant finding in depression (Corbett, 1980). Alternatively, the elderly individual who clings to work in a desperate way gives the nurse important clues about the fragile orientation of his or her self-concept and lack of acceptance of aging. Concretely, the nurse inquires what the patient's occupation was and when she or he retired. The patient is encouraged to expand on the information as seems appropriate based on the answers. It is important to focus on both positive aspects of the patient's work history as well as perhaps the more negative. The former gives the patient important recognition for accomplishments.

Physical Assessment

The depth of physical assessment performed by the nurse probably depends on the supports provided by the hospital. It is unnecessarily wearing to subject the patient to a separate physical exam by the attending physician, resident, and medical student as well as by the nurse. However, appropriate planning for nursing intervention with the elderly does require a somewhat specialized nursing assessment aimed at the patient's functional ability to participate in the milieu. In addition, the nurse can provide screening for physiological disorders that often present with an affective disorder.

In terms of functional physical assessment, the nurse is interested in primarily the patient's endurance: how far the patient is accustomed to walking each day, and how far he or she can walk in one effort without becoming fatigued or short of breath. The physical environment of a psychiatric unit may require far more exertion from the elderly patient just to walk from group therapy to his or her room and then to lunch than the patient is accustomed to. When the patient has obvious physical handicaps or a prosthesis that require more energy, it becomes more important to carefully assess the patient's lifestyle: how the patient copes at home, or what routine seems to work the best, or if the patient requires frequent breaks or a daily nap. Any of these findings indicate that some modifications of in-patient milieu may be necessary. The expectation of many psychiatric milieus is that the patient is active in group or other activity for the majority of the day. This expectation may be unrealistic for many elderly patients. The nurse and patient may need to prioritize and limit activity in order to avoid compounding a sense of failure for the depressed patient.

Sometimes a patient is not able to adequately describe the customary level of activity. In this case, the nurse may need to assess the patient's endurance on the unit as well as look to significant others for description.

Along with a description of physical activity, the patient also usually describes a pattern of rest. The nurse will want to assess whether a pattern of increased sleep has occurred and whether that sleep is restful. Depressed elderly frequently complain of increased sleep that is not restful. It is important to note signs of diural variation: depressed patients often feel slightly better as the day progresses and their cognitive function may even improve as well, but patients who have a greater degree of organicity usually decline in cognitive function over the course of the day. Here again, the patient's pattern of activity provides diagnostic clues as well as guidelines for reasonable milieu participation. Some expectations may be increased over time as the patient improves. The increase, however, should be gradual over the course of the hospital stay and correlated to clinical improvement rather than abruptly imposed. When the patient gives history of chronic disease, the nurse needs to note not only any physical findings associated with the patient's chronic illness but also what the patient's self-care regime has been. Here again, many patients have worked out a system that meets their needs far better than that health care providers could devise. To incorporate these regimes early on and make modifications in the milieu to accommodate them when reasonable avoids a great deal of tension and unnecessary focus away from therapeutic work.

It is also significant when a patient cannot identify a satisfactory regimen for an illness of long duration. While the implications for teaching and other intervention may seem clear, it is certainly just as important to examine the patient's psychological process in coping with his condition.

The nurse needs to determine whether the patient experiences any sensory losses common in the elderly. Hearing loss and changes in visual field, as well as decreased visual acuity, are frequently found. The impact of sensory losses are two-fold: these changes impact the patient's ability to participate in the milieu and may require nursing intervention to facilitate the patient's participation in groups. Sensory losses may also contribute to mental-status findings. Examples include a patient who appears paranoid but who actually experiences a hearing loss: it is common for this particular patient to feel that others are talking about him or her. A second example is a patient who initially appears withdrawn and detached, but becomes more animated and involved when sensory losses are accomodated.

In addition to the endurance capacity and sensory status of the patient, the nurse needs to be aware of any physical findings demanding immediate intervention. Self-neglect is often a part of the clinical picture for an elderly patient with an affective disorder. Since the nurse is often the first clinician to extensively assess the patient, she or he should be guided in assessment by what is seen occurring with the patient. Signs of dehydration, for example, should clue the nurse to quickly determine the patient's recent food and fluid intake. A lethargic patient with fluctuating level of consciousness demands assessment of vital signs, neurological and circulatory status, and drugs recently ingested. It may be that these findings demand nursing or medical intervention prior to further assessment.

The nurse needs to be generally aware of any physical findings indicative of a physical illness with an affective component. The importance of identifying an organic brain syndrome as part of the mental-status exam has already been discussed. Metastatic disease often includes depression as part of its clinical picture. Confusing the differential diagnosis even more are symptoms of weight loss, appetite loss, fatigue, and pain that may be present in both primary affective disorders and metastatic disease. Carcinoma of the pancreas is one malignancy particularly noted for causing depression early in its clinical course. Differentiating whether depression is the primary disorder or is secondary to another dysfunction can be difficult. The nurse can utilize family history to some extent for information regarding either situation. Any prior history of metastatic disease lends credence to the possibility of a recurrence. Additionally, any concurrent symptoms experienced by the patient may assist in developing a clinical picture, e.g., carcinoma of the pancreas classically includes a backache in addition to weight loss and depression.

Disorders of the endocrine system frequently cause depression. A patient with myxoedema may appear depressed but the clinical presentation includes muscle-wasting, weight loss, and atrial fibrillation. The patient with Cushing's syndrome might initially give the diagnostic impression of having an agitated depression or a depression with psychomotor retardation. Addison's disease may present with weight loss and decreased appetite, apathy, fatigue, and depression, in addition to postural hypotension and characteristic changes in skin pigmentation. Poor memory may also be present. Hyperparathyroidism may cause agitation, poor memory, and depression (Corbett, 1980).

Parkinson's disease can be mistaken for a primary depression due to the patient's fixed, flat facial expression and slowed movements, although more complete assessment for other characteristics of Parkinson's usually differentiates the two. Depression is frequently concomitant with Parkinson's disease, however, and demands concurrent treatment.

Malnutrition severe enough to cause a B_{12} or folate deficiency is unusual but such a deficiency can certainly cause depressive symptomatology. An electrolyte deficiency that mimics depression, particularly with malnutrition or physiological changes upsetting the body's regulation of such elements, is more common in the elderly. Indications of such problems are usually best screened and monitored by laboratory testing of serum electrolyte levels, although a thorough physical exam can provide some clues.

A relevant consideration in physical assessment is that an affective disorder may be present with nearly any chronic condition. Regardless of whether the affective disorder is caused by the chronic condition or not, psychiatric nursing considerations are present; e.g., one can ask if the patient is depressed with suicidal ideation. Age, as well as chronic illness, are judged to be risk factors for suicide. Determination of a discrete, physiologically based cause for an affective disorder does not preclude the necessity for treating the affective as well as the physiological components of the disease.

Drug History

Some drugs used in treatment of disorders common to the elderly can cause depression. This fact, plus the incidence of drug or alcohol abuse and misuse in the elderly, necessitate taking a drug history as part of the assessment process.

The nurse should ask the patient which drugs are taken, how frequently, in what dosage, and how helpful the patient feels the drugs are. If the patient does not mention over-the-counter drugs, the nurse needs to specifically inquire. If the patient identifies that a drug is not particularly helpful, the nurse can ask what other measures the patient takes for the condition, including offering an opening to discuss taking other than the prescribed dosage. If the assessment indicates a patient with memory loss who is responsible for self-medication, the nurse will want to ask how he or she organizes the medication regime. As a list of medications is developed, the nurse will need to be aware of any signs of overuse exhibited by the patient. He or she will also want to note any of the list that might precipitate a drug-induced affective disorder.

Antihypertensives are commonly implicated in depression. Reserpine is particularly culpable although propanolol and methyldopa may also cause a depression (Corbett, 1980). Tagamet given for gastric distress may contribute to an affective disorder.

L-Dopa can cause a severe depression in elderly patients with Parkinson's disease, making treatment extremely difficult. Digitalis toxicity may include depression or apathy as well as the more usual signs of nausea, vomiting, confusion, and changes in color vision. Steroids and anticancer drugs may also cause depression (Corbett, 1980).

Misuse of alcohol and minor tranquilizers can markedly affect mood. The nurse needs to take a tactful but careful history in this area. The frequency of alcoholism in the elderly may also indicate a futile attempt to address the despair of a depression.

Other Diagnostic Testing

In addition to assessment findings that can be concluded from talking with a patient, the nurse may find other diagnostic testing to be helpful. Although commonly initiated by the physician, a dexamethasone suppression test (DST), EEG, and computerized tomography of the brain (CT scan) provide helpful information to the nurse.

The DST is a protocol that evaluates dexamethasone suppression of serum cortisol. Depressed patients, including depressed elderly based on limited samples, do not exhibit the normal suppression of serum cortisol within 12 hours after ingestion of 1 mg of dexamethasone (Jenike, 1983). Because of the difficulty in diagnosing affective disorders in the elderly, DST can be a useful adjunct. Some clinical conditions do interfere with test results. These include alcoholism, anorexia nervosa, prolonged hemodialysis, Cushing's syndrome, malignancies with increased adrenocorticotropic hormone (ACTH) secretion, obesity, protein calorie malnutrition, renovascular hypertension, and uncontrolled diabetes mellitus. High-dose benzodiazepines, corticosteroids, and dextroamphetamine may increase dexamethsone suppression causing a false-negative result while phenytoin, barbiturates, and meprobamate may decrease the activity of dexamethasone yielding a false positive result (Jenike, 1983).

Other clinical applications for DST results have been suggested. Clinically depressed patients who do show DST suppression may respond to trycyclics that act by blocking reuptake of serotonin while those depressed patients who show a positive DST might be more appropriately treated with desipramine, for example, which blocks norepineprine reuptake (Brown et al., 1980). It has been tentatively identified that a return of normal DST suppression after nonsuppression and appropriate treatment could indicate resolution of a depression. This finding could therefore be a sign for gradual termination of drug therapy (Goldberg, 1980; Greden et al., 1980).

Grunhaus et al., (1983) examined the clinical assessment value of the DST and CT scan. They found their small sample of patients tended to divide into three groupings: patients with depressed mood, cognitive impairment, abnormal DST results, and normal CT scans were likely to have depressive psuedodementia; patients with depressed mood, cognitive impairment, and abnormal DST and CT scan tended to be depressed as well as organic; the "truely demented" patients had a normal DST results and an abnormal CT scan. Although the investigators point out the need for further study, the diagnostic assistance of the DST and CT scan are indicated.

INTERVENTIONS

Interventions for elderly patients hospitalized with a diagnosis of depression are based on data obtained in the initial assessment. Their modification will take place because of time restraints, change in patient status, and various structures present in the hospital. As hospital stays get shorter, time becomes a factor in implementing the most effective combination of treatment modalities. Some of the more common modalities available to nurses include milieu therapy (i.e., the therapeutic community), individual therapy, group therapy, family counseling, and adjunct treatment modalities encompassing psychopharmcological and ECT.

The therapeutic community represents one of the major structures encountered in the hospital setting. Emphasis is placed on interpersonal aspects of the patient's functioning. The effectiveness depends to a large extent on the social environment created by the milieu. The therapeutic community allows the patient to have a more active role in self-therapy and the therapy of others. The nurse supports open communication with staff and other patients, allowing the patient to gain insight into the maladaptive behaviors that influenced hospitalization.

For the depressed elderly person, the structure of a therapeutic community may need certain modifications to allow positive outcomes. Initial entry into the milieu may require a much more gradual course. The nurse must recognize the marked differences in the milieu from the patient's home environment. For many elderly people living alone for several years, the changes can be drastic. For instance, the patients may be accustomed to a small living space and minimal contact with other people. The new milieu may create an overload of stimuli for the individual. If the patient population includes a mix of both young and old, nurses need to identify the elderly patient's comfort level and the milieu's response to his or her presence. They should not anticipate conflict between younger and older patients. Anxiety can more likely be a result of the elderly patient's inexperience and fear of the unknown. The nurse, therefore, should assist the patient in entering the system, keeping in mind individual needs for privacy and quiet. Group activities may be limited by such realities as sensory deficits and physical disabilities. For example, ambulating the distance of the hallway in a walker may be a major obstacle to participation in milieu therapy.

To counteract the elderly depressed patient's feelings of worthlessness and hopelessness nurses must apply some basic skills, such as fostering independence to allow the individual to feel some sense of control. They facilitate this process by encouraging the patient to participate in decision making regarding his or her own care. Self-esteem may be enhanced by giving the individual the opportunity to select clothes for the day, and foods preferred for meals. Nurses should consider the patient's selection of unit activities as well as personal quiet time when planning a day-to-day treatment regime.

Certain aids may be useful in communicating with the elderly. A slower response time for the elderly should be kept in mind. Listening may be a more tedious task for the nurse but it serves as an essential component of interventions. It is important to allow sufficient time for the elderly person to express thoughts and feelings. If attempts are made to speed up the communication process, anxiety may force the patient to omit or pass over important details. In an attempt to be understood, the elderly person may instead feel humiliated and even more worthless.

One-to-one therapeutic interventions may be required to meet basic physical needs. Vegetative symptoms that include an inability to care for basic bodily needs such as eating, sleeping, and grooming, should be addressed. Improvement in cognitive functioning usually follows an improvement in ability to meet basic bodily needs. The patient may then become part of a higher level of individual therapy with the nurse.

In some cases, one-to-one talk therapy is an appropriate modality for hospitalized patients. Certain considerations are indicated for the nurse involved in such treatment with the elderly patient. First, consider how receptive the patient is toward this approach, and what goals are feasible for that patient. Success of a one-to-one talk therapy depends on how realistic and attainable the goals are as well as the motivation for goal achievement on the part of the patient and nurse therapist.

Many elderly persons reject a diagnosis of depression. For some, it many hold special meaning counter to deep-seated values. The elderly person may react to the stigma attached to the label of mental illness as well as memories of unacceptable treatment used for patients in the past. This response may increase the individual's sense of hopelessness. Goals for talk therapy, therefore, should be set to assist these patients in understanding and accepting their present depressed state. By educating the patient about newer and safer treatments for depression, nurses can help dispel misconceptions. Withdrawn and isolative patients are not necessarily unresponsive to one-to-one talk therapies. Simple goals, such as returning a greeting in the hallway, or being able to sit in the presence of the nurse for increasing amounts of time, can be starting places for one-to-one talk therapies. Elderly patients with multiple somatic complaints may be more than eager to discuss them within this format. Even though it is a tedious task to redirect the somatic patient to other issues and topics, a discussion of anything beyond somatic complaints for these patients may be a goal well-achieved.

Caution also must be considered in the use of insight-oriented talk-therapy. Although gaining insight into one's depression may be beneficial, at the same time it can be devastating. For the elderly person the realities that surround the depression may become a frightening experience. So, timing should be considered in encouraging the elderly patient to examine her or his own depression in any depth. A severly depressed person, however, may not be capable of developing insight because of an inability to concentrate. Other factors, such as a lack of sleep and poor food intake contribute to the situation. Unsuccessful efforts toward gaining insight will likely increase the patient's sense of failure and hopelessness.

Another treatment modality accessible to the nurse is group therapy. Group therapies for elderly depressed individuals can be especially useful to reinforce adaptive behavior, improve communication and social skills, and provide support. As a group leader, the nurse faces the task of facilitating positive outcome for the members. He or she assumes a supportive, empathetic role in providing a healthy environment for effective group work to occur. Elderly persons, unlike their younger counterparts, are more apt to have multiple problems including social, physical, and mental disabilities. The group leaders need to facilitate optimum hearing, vision, and understanding for each group member. A slower pace for the group may be necessary, to allow adequate time for listening and responding to others in a meaningful way. Sensory deficits may require keeping the group smaller with members sitting closer together.

The elderly depressed individual may resist group work, especially with exposure to other depressed elderly people. He may even wonder, "How can talking in a group of depressed older people possibly help me?" The leader can facilitate the group by discussing the potential relief effect that exists in listening to another person expressing concerns similar to their own. By discovering similarities and sharing experiences and feelings, group members may feel less isolated and alone in their depression. By revealing the potential benefits of interacting with others in group the nurse can enhance the process and "get the group going."

Clear messages about group rules and goals enhance the beginning group. Elderly individuals may need frequent reminders about time, place, and length of group meetings. The nurse can overcome many of the resistances to attending group by taking extra time before each group meeting to invite members individually.

Reminiscing can be a useful tool in the group's work. Group creates a rich arena for the individual to re-experience the past through the lives of others. Therefore, the setting can be a natural place for reminiscing to evolve. Group members can experience a bolstering of their self-esteem, as well as a higher level of group cohesion through reminiscing. An adaptive process occurs when the elderly person reminisces past-life experiences. The process can assist the older individual in feeling worthwhile in life as well as coping with the painful realities of her or his present life. Coping means that the elderly individual remembers having adaptive coping abilities and a strong self-concept.

The elderly patient is not the only one to suffer in the face of depression. Family members are a part of the crisis, including suffering the effects of the depression with which their elderly family member is afflicted. Therefore, another treatment modality available to nursing intervention includes counseling the family of the hospitalized elderly patient. The impact of such counseling can result in final decisions about the future of the elderly family member.

An elderly parent suffering from depressive symptoms may present him- or herself as a weak force against a unified group of siblings who are determined that "something must be done." The nurse may find herself unable to influence or contest the family's decision. Interventions with the family can be modified by focusing on a realistic problem, such as how the patient can be managed after discharge. Interventions might include helping the family recognize the patient's level of functioning and exploring ways to deal with that level of functioning after discharge. By visiting in the hospital the family can actually visualize and assist in patient care. This may be the best way to help family members see the situation realistically.

Pathology may exist in the family's functioning, such as the "unspoken rules" that exist and influence family decisions. Family rules may include, "We never allow ourselves to be emotional", or, "Father always has the last word." Usually, it is unrealistic to expect to change the family system, although these bits of assessment data can be useful in deciding what is realistic to work on with the family.

Hopelessness and desperation create a helpless atmosphere in which the family must work. Empathy on the part of the nurse can be utilized to acknowledge the family's feeling of hopelessness. The nurse can act as a barometer and a sounding board for the expression of emotional tension. Arguing with the family or telling them what to do is useless and stifles any successful problem solving that the family may be able to do on its own.

Identifying the patient's strongest support system in the family can be useful. This person may ultimately feel a great deal of pressure and responsibility in assuming the care-taker role for the patient. By offering support to this family member the nurse has a vehicle to assess the willingness as well as ability of this individual to actually take on the care-taker role. Also, helping this family member to speak out in family counseling meetings can prevent a poor outcome for the patient.

Adjunct treatment modalities, including the use of electroconvulsive therapy and medications are frequently a major mode of intervention for the depressed elderly person. The nurse's attitude about the use of medication and ECT can influence the patient's response. Anxiety about side-effects and potential complications may be transmitted to the patient even when the nurse makes a conscious effort to conceal them.

Changes in normal body functioning occur with aging. Generally, body systems slow down and are not as efficient. Therefore, toxicity and cumulative effects from drugs are suspect in the elderly. Even though the elderly pose certain limitations in the use of medications it should not impede treatment for depressive symptomatology. When drug treatment is planned, individualized and monitored, its use can be justified; e.g., severely depressed individuals who are anorectic or suicidal often times remain unchanged until given antidepressants or ECT.

Tricyclic antidepressants remain the treatment of choice for many depressions in the elderly. A variety of medications under the tricyclic label allow for selection and adjustment according to depressive symptoms. Two major classes of tricyclics—sedating and nonsedating—will be considered. The nonsedating tricyclics include protriptyline, desipramine and imipramine. The elderly who experience depressions with psychomotor retardation are more often successfully treated with nonsedating tricyclics. The sedating tricyclics are indicated for depressions that present with hyperactivity and agitation. They include doxepin, amitriptyline, and nortriptyline.

Postural hypotension, a troublesome side effect, is a concern because of the risk of falls, transient ischemic attacks, and strokes. Because of these hypotensive effects, the use of tricyclics should only be advised for patients with adequate cardiac functioning. To avoid orthostatic hypotensive episodes, the elderly patient should be directed to rise more slowly than usual from prone or sitting positions. This effect usually resolves itself after the drug treatment progresses.

Anticholinergic side effects may not be a concern for younger adults but pose a serious problem for the elderly; e.g., a dry mouth caused by these drugs may create a substantial problem for the many elderly individuals who wear dentures. Constipation, blurred vision, urinary retention, and mental confusion that occur in many elderly people not taking tricyclics may become compounded after starting drug treatment.

Therapeutic lag-time for the tricyclic antidepressants is often 3-4 weeks, to allow the drug to reach adequate blood levels. The elderly depressed patient, who will likely have difficulty identifying the changes resulting from drug therapy, may be discouraged by the delay in symptom relief. The nurse can be helpful by observing and reporting any objective improvements that may indicate the onset of symptom relief.

The use of monoamine oxidase (MAO) inhibitors are often avoided in the elderly. The danger of hypertensive side effects associated with combinations of MAO inhibitors and certain foods or medications warrant cautiousness in their use. Dietary restrictions while the patient is in the hospital, frequently need the nurse's attention because the depressed individual may not cognitively be able to make appropriate food selections. As depressive symptoms decrease and cognitive functioning improves, the patient may be able to independently restrict his or her diet safely. Planning and teaching for safe medication use after discharge are important aspects of patient care. The family may need to be a part of the discharge planning process, especially if the elder family member has impaired functioning.

In recent literature the MAO inhibitors are gaining support, especially with resistant geriatric depressions. The rationale for their efficacy is based on the finding that MAO activity increases in the body with aging. This suggests that the MAO inhibitors may be more effective for some geriatric depressions. Those that support the use of MAO inhibitors also suggest that there is less problem with sedation and the anticholinergic side effects that normally occur with the use of tricyclics.

Electroconvulsive therapy (ECT) is a safe alternative for the endogenously depressed elderly person. It remains the treatment of choice when antidepressant medications are unsuccessful or contraindicated for medical reasons. In fact, when one looks at the complications and side effects of medication use in the elderly the consideration of ECT seems to be a relatively safe alternative. Also, in view of the delayed therapeutic response of medication use, the high-risk suicidal or anorectic patient may need a more immediate therapeutic outcome that can be provided by ECT. In these high-risk patients, the presence of dementia should not avert treatment. Even though ECT is usually always effective the risk of relapse is high. The use of maintenance antidepressant medications can decrease the danger of relapse (Corbett, 1980).

Fear of loss of consciousness and amnesia following treatment may create high anxiety in elderly patients anticipating ECT. The nurse can assess and intervene with the elderly patient's knowledge of ECT. Misconceptions about the use of ECT should be clarified. A careful explanation of the procedure including post-ECT nursing care can reduce unrealistic fears. It also may be useful to utilize other patients receiving ECT to offer support to the patient facing ECT for the first time.

THE SUICIDAL ELDERLY PATIENT

The elderly are more at risk for carrying out successful suicides than younger individuals. Suicide can be thought of as a rational act for some elderly individuals. Losses are a prominent feature, including loss of job and status as well as failing body functioning. An elderly retired male who is suffering from a costly terminal illness may rationalize suicide. It assists him to gain control of the demise he is slowly facing and also leaves his widow in a more sound financial situation.

The suicides that are associated with depressive illness and result in hospitalization are more likely to be prevented. The nurse's skill in assessment and intervention on the psychiatric unit are keys to providing a safe environment for the suicidal patient. A patient who is preoccupied with suicidal thought needs close observation and a structured environment. Both can be provided in the hospital setting. Openly discussing the topic of suicide is important with the verbal patient. One-to-one meetings with the nurse as well as group therapies can be useful. The acutely suicidal elderly patient requires aggressive intervention that may include one-to-one monitoring, physical restraint, and/or the consideration of emergency ECT.

The passively suicidal elderly patient may be more difficult to identify and intervene with. These patients require the same degree of attention and contact with the nurse. Behaviors may be identified that have self-destructive intentions. For example, a passive suicidal elderly person may refuse food or medications. A careful assessment is required in determining self-destructive behaviors, as some behaviors may be mislabelled as self-destructive. Organic changes that create variations in behavior can appear to have self-destructive qualities. To label a patient that climbs out of a wheelchair and falls as self-destructive requires consideration of the behaviors intent. What is the message being sent by the patient's behavior? Has the behavior change occurred recently? Are there other clues of change to a self-destructive mode? Answers to these questions can assist the nurse to intervene and provide the appropriate protective environment.

THE NURSE–PATIENT RELATIONSHIP

The depressed elderly patient admitted to the hospital presents a particularly gloomy picture for the nurse. Elderly patients may range anywhere from 20-to 60-years-older than nursing staff. The patient is not only "old" but may be despondent, hopeless, and unable to care for himself. Difficulty may arise in accepting the dependent nature of the depressed older person. The nurse's empathy and understanding are challenged as basic physiological and safety needs become a priority for patient care.

Other troublesome aspects of caring for the depressed elderly person may stem from complicating factors that the patient brings to the hospital. Physical illness such as heart disease, diabetes, or Parkinson's disease will modify possible nursing interventions. Also, varying degrees of dementia complicate the depressive picture and limit the potentials for positive outcome by way of the nurse-patient relationship.

Various treatments ordered during the hospital stay also influence the nurse-patient relationship. ECT may be indicated due to life threatening symptoms or disease processes. The resulting amnesia frequently limit or postpone the continuity of the nurse–patient relationship. As a result, more time will be spent monitoring recovery and reacquainting the patient to his immediate environment. The use of pharmacotherapy for the hospitalized depressed elderly patient also influences the nurse–patient relationship.

With progress in understanding depression and neurotransmitters in the body, many new drugs and drug combinations are being used. The nurse is challenged to confront new and emergent situations with elderly patients receiving drug therapies. The hospital stay often becomes the testing ground for monitoring effectiveness and side effects of various drug treatments. Therefore, the nurse may feel cast into a role of doling out medication, observing for effectiveness, and maintaining safety in the case of adverse side effects.

The nurse–patient relationship with the hospitalized, depressed elderly person seems limited in many ways. Short hospital stays, severity of illness, and treatment issues, along with the nurse's attitude about caring for a dependent elderly person all become restricting factors. Positive outcome by way of a therapeutic nurse–patient relationship may be an unrealistic goal for the nurse to consider.

In spite of the realistic limitations, nursing intervention with the elderly in an in-patient psychiatric milieu contributes to significant patient improvement. The multiple concerns of the patient require thorough and careful assessment as well as judicious incorporation of the findings into the overall plan of care. The nurse may find it necessary to modify milieu expectations for the patient in order to develop a realistic plan that meets the patient's clinical need for psychiatric nursing intervention while allowing for physical and functional limitations.

REFERENCES

Brown, W. A., Harir, R. J., & Qualls, C. B. (1980). Dexamethsone suppression that identifies subtypes of depression which respond to different antidepressants. *Lancet, 1*(8174), 928.

Burnside, I. M. (1981). *Nursing and the aged.* New York: McGraw-Hill.

Butler, R. N. (1963). The life review: An interpretation of reminiscence in the aged. *Psychiatry, 26*(1), 65–76.

Corbett, L. (1980). *The recognition of disguised depressive illness and the pharmacologic treatment of depression in the elderly.* Chicago; Rush University, unpublished manuscript.

Ebersole, P., & Hess, P. (1981). *Toward healthy aging: Human needs and nursing response.* St. Louis: C. V. Mosby.

Frank, J. D. (1974). *Persuasion and healing* (Rev. ed.). New York: Schocken Books.

Goldberg, I. K. (1980). Dexamethasone suppression test as indicator of safe withdrawal of antidepressant therapy. *Lancet, 1*(8164), 376.

Greden, J. F., Albala, A. A., Haskett, R. F., James, N. M., Goodman, L., Steiner, M., & Carroll, B. J. (1980). Normalization of dexamethasone suppression test: A laboratory index of recovery from endogenous depression. *Biological Psychiatry, 15*(3), 449–458.

Grunhaus, L., Dilsaver, S., Greden, J. F., & Carroll, B. J. (1983). Depressive pseudodementia: A suggested diagnostic profile. *Biological Psychiatry, 18*(2), 215–225.

Jenike, M. A. (1983). Dexamethasone suppression test as a clinical aid in elderly depressed patients. *Journal of American Geriatrics Society, 31*(1), 45–48.

Johnson, C. W., Snibbe, J. R., & Evans, L. A. (1975). *Basic psychopathology: A programmed text.* New York: Spectrum Publications.

Nelson, F. L., & Farberow, N. L. (1976). Indirect suicide in the elderly chronically ill patient. In K. Anchte and J. Lonnquist (Eds.), *Suicide research.* Helsinki: Psychiatria Fennica Supplement.

Pfeiffer, E. (1975). A short portable mental status questionnaire for the assessment of organic brain deficit in elderly patients. *Journal of American Geriatrics Society, 23*(10), 433–441.

Simos, B. G. (1979). *A time to grieve: Loss as a universal human experience.* New York: Family Service Association of America.

Smyer, M., Hofland, B., & Jonas, E. (1979). Validity study of the short portable mental status questionnaire for the elderly. *Journal of the American Geriatrics Society, 27*(6), 263–269.

Verwoerdt, A. (1981). *Clinical geropsychiatry* (2nd ed.). Baltimore: Williams and Wilkins.

Wolanin, M. O. & Phillips, L. R. (1981). *Confusion: prevention and care.* St. Louis: C. V. Mosby.

SUGGESTED READINGS

Atchley, R. C. (1982). The aging self. *Psychotherapy: Theory, Research, and Practice, 19*(4), 388–397.

Blau, D., & Berezin, M. A. (1982). Neuroses and character disorder. *Journal of Geriatric Psychiatry, 15*(1), 55–97.

Blazer, D. (1983). The epidemiology of late life depression. *Journal of the American Geriatrics Society, 30*(9), 587–593.

Brink, T. L. (1982). Geriatric depression and hypochondriasis: Incidence, interaction, assessment, and treatment. *Psychotherapy: Theory, Research, and Practice, 19*(4), 506–511.

Brown, R., Sweeney, J., Frances, A., Kocsis, J. H., & Loutsch, E. (1983). Age as a predictor of treatment response in endogenous depression. *Journal of Clinical Psychopharmacology, 3*(3), 176–178.

Burnside, I. M. (1969). Group work among the aged. *Nursing Outlook, 17*(6), 68–71.

Butler, R. N. (1960). Intensive psychotherapy for the hospitalized aged. *Geriatrics, 15*(9), 644–653.

Cavanaugh, S., & Wettstein, R. M. (1983). The relationship between severity of depression, cognitive dysfunction, and age in medical in-patients. *American Journal of Psychiatry, 140*(4), 495–496.

de Figueiredo, J. M., & Frank, J. D. (1982). Subjective incompetence, the clinical hallmark of demoralization. *Comprehensive Psychiatry, 23*(4), 353–363.

Dellefield, K., & Miller, J. (1982). Psychotropic drugs and the elderly patient. *Nursing Clinics of North America, 17*(2), 303–318.

Emery, G., & Lesher, E. (1982). Treatment of depression in older adults: Personality considerations. *Psychotherapy: Theory, Research and Practice, 19*(4), 500–505.

Epstein, L. J. (1976). Symposium on age differentiation in depressive illness. *Journal of Gerontology, 31*(3), 278–282.

Fann, W. E. (1976). Pharmacotherapy in older depressed patients. *Journal of Gerontology, 31*(3), 304–310.

Fraser, R. M., & Glass, I. B. (1978). Recovery from ECT in elderly patients. *British Journal of Psychiatry, 133*, 524–528.

Gaspar, D., & Samarsinghe, L. A. (1982). ECT in psychogeriatric practice—A study of risk factors, indications and outcome. *Comprehensive Psychiatry, 23*(4), 170–175.

Georgotas, A., Friedman, E., McCarthy, M., Mann, J., Krakowski, M., Siegel, R., & Ferris, S. (1983). Resistant geriatric depressions and therapeutic response to monamine oxidase inhibitors. *Biological Psychiatry, 18*(2), 195–205.

Grunhaus, L., Dilsaver, S., Greden, J. F., & Carroll, B. J. (1983). Depressive pseudodementia: A suggested diagnostic profile. *Biological Psychiatry, 18*(2), 215–225.

Hayes, J. E. (1982). Normal changes in aging and nursing implications of drug therapy. *Nursing Clinics of North America, 17*(2), 253–262.

Hirshfeld, M. J. (1977). Nursing care of the cognitively impaired aged. In C. Eisdorfer & R. O. Friedel (Eds.), *Cognitive and emotional disturbance in the elderly* (pp. 121–128). Chicago: Year Book Medical Publishers.

Jarvik, L. F., Read, S. L., Mintz, J., & Neshkes, R. E. (1983). Pretreatment orthostatic hypotension in the geriatric depression: Predictor of response to imipramine and doxepin. *Journal of Clinical Psychopharmacology, 3*(6), 368–372.

Jenike, M. A. (1983). Dexamethasone suppression test as a clinical aid in elderly depressed patients. *Journal of American Geriatrics Society, 31*(1), 45–48.

Knesevich, J. W., Martin, R. L., Berg, L., & Danziger, W. (1983). Preliminary report on affective symptoms in the early stages of senile dementia of the Alzheimer type. *American Journal of Psychiatry, 140*(2), 233–235.

Kramer, B. A. (1982). Depressive pseudodementia. *Comprehensive Psychiatry, 23*(6), 538–544.

Lakin, M., Oppenheimer, B., & Bremer, J. (1982). A note on old and young in helping groups. *Psychotherapy: Theory, Research and Practice, 19*(4), 444–454.

Lancaster, J. (1981). Maximizing psychological adaptation in an aging population. *Topics in Clinical Nursing, 3*(1), 31–43.

Lazarus, L. W. (1976). A program for the elderly at a private psychiatric hospital. *The Gerontologist, 16*(2), 125–131.

Lewis, J. M., & Johansen, K. H. (1982). Resistances to psychotherapy with the elderly. *American Journal of Psychotherapy, 36*(4), 497–504.

Lewis, M. I., & Butler, R. N. (1974). Life-review therapy: Putting memories to work in individual and group psychotherapy. *Geriatrics, 29*(11), 165–173.

Lippman, S. (1983). Drug therapy for depression in the elderly. *Postgraduate Medicine, 73*(1), 159–169.

Lipton, M. A. (1976). Age differentiation in depression: Biochemical aspects. *Journal of Gerontology, 31*(3), 293–299.

Mendlewicz, J. (1976). The age factor in depressive illness: Some genetic considerations. *Journal of Gerontology, 31*(3), 300–303.

Murrell, S. A., Himmelfarb, S., & Wright, K. (1983). Prevalence of depression and its correlates in older adults. *American Journal of Epidemiology, 117*(2), 173–185.

Pedder, J. R. (1982). Failure to mourn and melancholia. *British Journal of Psychiatry, 141*, 329–337.

Pitt, B. (1982). The psychogeriatric patient. In B. Pitt, (Ed.) *Psychogeriatrics: An introduction to the psychiatry of old age* (2nd ed.). Edinburgh: Churchill Livingstone.

Rabins, P. V. (1982). Psychopathology of Parkinson's disease. *Comprehensive Psychiatry, 23*(5), 421–429.

Sandler, Anne-Marie. (1982). Psychoanalysis and psychoanalytic psychotherapy of the older patient. *Journal of Geriatric Psychiatry, 15*(1), 11–32.

Van Praag, H. M. (1982). The significance of biological factors in the diagnosis of depressions: I. Biochemical variables. *Comprehensive Psychiatry, 23*(2), 124–135.

Vickers, R. (1976). The therapeutic milieu and the older depressed patient. *Journal of Gerontology, 31*(3), 314–317.

Weinberg, J. (1979). Of slings and arrows and outrageous fortune. *The American Journal of Psychoanalysis, 19*(3), 195–210.

Wells, C. E. (1979). Pseudodementia. *American Journal of Psychiatry, 136*(7), 895–900.

Yalom, I. D., & Terrazas, F. (1968). Group therapy for psychotic elderly patients. *American Journal of Nursing, 68*(8), 1690–1694.

Yesavage, J. A., & Karasu, T. B. (1982). Psychotherapy with elderly patients. *American Journal of Psychotherapy, 36*(1), 41–55.

	Individualizing Antidepressant Therapies
12	**Kathryn Gleason Cook**

For most of the past 25 years, biochemical treatment of depression has been anchored by the use of a single broad-spectrum tricyclic antidepressant (TCA), such as imipramine or amitriptyline, bringing relief to thousands, and meanwhile fostering simplistic thinking among clinicians about cause and treatment of affective disorders. More recently, however, increasingly complex antidepressant combinations have been formulated to the extent that, among some inpatient populations, it is relatively uncommon to find patients treated with single-drug regimens. At the same time, highly individualized antidepressant protocols are being designed for specific subcategories of the depressed population. Nursing assessments can make a major contribution to the development, selection, and management of complex therapeutic combinations in addition to the traditional role nurses have performed in medication administration.

DEVELOPMENT OF INDIVIDUALIZED THERAPIES

At least four factors in contemporary biological psychiatry have fostered the trend toward increasing individualization of antidepressant therapies. A significant impetus has been the identification of depressive syndromes refractory or resistant to simple TCA treatment. In early systematic reviews of TCA efficacy (Davis, 1976; Morris & Beck, 1974), some 70–75% of depressed patients were thought to respond satisfactorily to traditional protocols, but later analyses have set the figure as low as 60% (Avery & Winokur, 1977; Fink, 1978; Stern et al., 1980; Zarifian & Rigal, 1982), leaving a substantial number of persons without symptomatic relief. That such a subpopulation exists is no surprise to experienced clinicians familiar with the recidivism of depression. In some instances, these are individuals who have achieved some degree of improvement with TCAs, but either failed to maintain that improvement (suffering a relapse), or did not achieve a degree of clinical improvement to free them from the disabling effects of affective disorder. Such patients represent a diverse diagnostic category, lacking clear definition and defying analysis as to the origin of their treatment resistance. Nonetheless, these people do share a commonality of having disabling, even life-threatening depressive symptomatology, and poignantly but urgently presenting clinicians with the need to create and test new therapeutic regimens.

Traditional TCA therapies have become less desirable as an ever-growing population of elderly depressives is identified and treated. Variable metabolic effects in the elderly, along with an increased propensity to develop side effects and vulnerability for their sequelae (Klein et al., 1980), necessitate modifications in dosage regimens, sometimes compromising the ability to achieve therapeutic plasma levels. For this group, a broad-spectrum TCA may not only fail to produce clinical improvement, but may directly or indirectly evoke other health problems, such as falls, urinary difficulties, or cardiac arrhythmias. At the same time, elderly depressives often present clinical symptomatology significantly different from that of younger adults. Frank agitation is often a concomitant of depression in the elderly to the extent that it requires special medication management, sometimes compromising the usual TCA regimen.

Similarly, the emergence of significant numbers of persons who are medically ill, but also have depressive symptomatology requiring vigorous biological intervention, has made modifications in traditional approaches mandatory. Persons with pre-existing cardiac conditions, glaucoma, and benign prostatic hypertrophy represent a small percentage of the individuals who are likely to experience significant worsening of their medical conditions in response to traditional TCA therapies. Toxic effects of TCAs are well-documented (Cassem, 1982; Jefferson, 1975; Preskorn & Irwin, 1982) and can easily be developed in a variety of other illnesses as well, either as a result of the medical condition itself or TCA-drug interactions. The morbidity associated with TCA-induced cardiotoxicity alone has compelled the development of newer agents with fewer such side effects.

Availability of larger numbers of agents having antidepressant effects, along with the evolution of increasingly complex models of affective disorders, have irrevocably altered conservative TCA regimens. More detailed explication of synaptic transmission processes in catecholamine and indolamine systems—from neurotransmitter synthesis through receptor-blockade—has made possible additional substances with the potential for clinical antidepressant effects that are derived from their activity in central nervous system synapses (Ananth, 1983). Recognition of differences between short- and long-term effects of antidepressant medications (Heninger et al., 1983; Oswald et al., 1972) has led to the exploration of other mechanisms implicated in the central effects of affective disorder and subsequently, to the discovery of the antidepressant efficacy of still other substances, such as lithium. Consideration of alternative hypotheses of affective disorders (Sabelli & Mosnaim, 1974) has resulted in preliminary investigations of additional nontraditional antidepressant treatment strategies (Sabelli et al., 1983a). Finally, investigations of the clinical efficacy of substances known to have specific neurochemical activity, but heretofore not recognized as antidepressants, have led to the discovery of the "second-generation antidepressants" (Shopsin, 1980), many of which are not yet released for clinical use. As a result of these interacting forces, the number of available antidepressants has grown considerably, but more importantly, there has been a tactical change in antidepressant therapy constituting a separate clinical technology.

TECHNOLOGY OF INDIVIDUALIZED THERAPIES

Renewed use of MAO inhibitors. Subsequent to the identification of a significant group of patients who did not demonstrate therapeutic response to TCAs, psychiatrists began to re-examine the utility of monoamine oxidase inhibitors (MAOIs), a group that had largely fallen into disrepute because of side-effects or limited clinical results (Klerman, 1978; Richelson, 1982). As a result, MAOIs are now used more frequently after unsuccessful TCA trials, in combination with TCAs or other drugs, and sometimes preferentially for some diagnostic subtypes such as *atypical* depression (Moreines & Gold, 1984; Robinson et al., 1973). Most nurses have some familiarity with MAOIs and their difficulties, especially the hypertensive episodes they can precipitate when certain foods or drugs are ingested. The clinical literature is replete with descriptions of those interactive effects, lists of likely offenders, and protocols for management (Kline & Cooper, 1980; Moreines & Gold, 1984; Schoonover, 1983). However, two other effects of MAOIs have received relatively less attention in the clinical literature, yet have significant implications for nursing practice.

The first, orthostatic hypotension, is particularly significant because it is the primary reason patients stop treatment, fail to comply, or suffer serious sequelae from falls and other injuries (Richelson, 1982). Unlike the orthostatic hypotension associated with TCAs, MAOI-induced hypotension occurs much later in therapy, frequently in the third, fourth, or fifth weeks of treatment. Once established, it is not likely to spontaneously remit and will require some type of management. Exercise, caffeine, and oral fludrocortisone have all been recommended to counteract MAOI-induced orthostatic hypotension (Kline & Cooper, 1980; Moreines & Gold, 1984). Certainly, patients need to be prepared for the possibility of hypotensive changes and informed of the actions they can take to decrease the likelihood of resultant injury. It is possible that persons who are apt to develop orthostatic hypotension can be identified prior to beginning treatment by postural changes they have demonstrated previously (Glassman et al., 1979). Clearly, persons who have pre-existing orthostatic changes should be identified as being at risk for further MAOI-related hypotensive changes.

An aside regarding blood pressure measurement in psychiatric nursing seems appropriate at this point. Contrary to prevailing attitudes in many settings, blood pressure measurement is not a ritualistic, casual activity. Rather, it requires skill, strict adherence to guidelines, such as those designed by the American Heart Association (Bates, 1983), and clinical expertise in interpretation of objective results as compared with reported symptomatology. Accurate baseline data is absolutely critical to the identification of serious side effects and ultimately, perhaps success of the regimen itself.

Another troublesome effect of MAOIs is the potential for addiction or tolerance in at least some patients. MAOIs are closely related to the amphetamines, and produce in a few individuals, a euphoriant effect, or "rush," similar to that associated with amphetamines (Shopsin & Kline, 1976). Euphoriant and antidepressant effects of MAOIs are distinctly different and can be clinically separated as well. Euphoriant effects appear about one hour after each MAOI dose, have clearly identifiable pleasant qualities for the individual who may label them as a "rush" or "buzz" in some mild form. These effects last for a couple of hours, and gradually dissipate. Over a period of weeks, the patient requires larger and larger amounts of MAOI to achieve these effects, producing an addictive syndrome that can lead to life-threatening overdosages (Kline & Cooper, 1980). Careful observation of patients using MAOIs for the first time, especially if there is indication of substance-abusing histories can be instrumental in identifying potential MAOI abuse.

Another relatively recent development is the use of platelet assay to monitor MAOI therapy. Platelets contain significant amounts of Type B MAO, similar to that found in the central nervous system and accurately reflecting the central inhibition induced by MAOIs (Davidson et al., 1978). These qualities make platelet MAO activity a valid biological marker of the progress of MAOI therapy. A usual protocol is to measure baseline platelet MAO activity prior to starting therapy, followed by serial measurements after three or four weeks (Moreines & Gold, 1984). Patients who achieve 80% platelet MAO inhibition are much more likely to experience significant clinical improvement (Raft et al.,1981; Robinson et al., 1978) than those who fail to reach adequate inhibition

(Ravaris et al., 1976). Dosage requirements will be adjusted using a combination of assay results and clinical data.

Selection of specific TCA.   A difficult decision confronting clinicians is selection of the initial TCA with which to treat a depressed patient. Ideally, it would be possible to expertly match the biological parameters of a patient with a TCA having the greatest probability of producing a therapeutic response, and then use serial measurements to determine the most efficacious dosage for all phases of treatment. In the absence of such a system, there are biological markers that offer some guidance and, when taken in series, constitute a very rough decision tree for selection of specific TCA therapy.

One such marker, the dexamethasone suppression test (DST), is a popular and valuable tool for identification of depressed individuals (*nonsuppressors*) who are candidates for biochemical therapy (Carroll et al., 1976). Despite early hopes that the DST would function as a highly predictive biological marker directing treatment strategy (Coryell, 1982), no evidence has been identified that nonsuppression on the DST is predictive of a positive response to any specific TCA (Carroll, 1984; Fraser, 1983). In some depressed patients treated bio-chemically, normalization of the DST will occur before positive clinical re-sponses are obtained (Albala et al., 1981), but other patients improve clinically while remaining as DST nonsuppressors (Carroll, 1982). Finally, in patients with significant symtomatology, normal DST results do not preclude appropriate use of antidepressant therapies (Carroll, 1982).

Stimulant-challenge tests have been more successful in anticipating specific TCA responses. Dextro-amphetamine (Fawcett & Siomopoulos, 1971; Fawcett et al., 1972; Maas et al., 1972; Van Kammen & Murphy, 1978) or methylpheni-date (Brown & Brawley, 1983; Sabelli et al., 1983b), administered in similar protocols, produce behavioral changes predictive of TCA-responsiveness in the third or fourth week of therapy. Patients experiencing a positive response to stimulant challenge are thought to respond best to imipramine or desipramine, while those who do not have a positive response are more likely to respond to amitriptyline or nortriptyline. While these results suggest TCA selection, they are not absolutely predictive (Ettigi et al., 1983; Sabelli et al., 1983b; Van Kammen & Murphy, 1978).

Most clearly evident 1½–2 hours after test-dose administration, a positive response consists of a marked improvement in mood, affect, and motor behavior that may manifest itself in significant changes in activities of daily living. Per-sonal appearance, responsiveness to environment and social interaction may all show brief, but significant improvement. In a clearly positive response, patients can actively describe their subjective sense of improvement. Clearly negative responses are also easily identifiable; significant irritability, increasing agitation (Kiloh et al., 1974), and sometimes even frank irascibility develop just as quickly and last for a similar time course as does the positive response. Others simply do not experience any change in symptomatology subsequent to stimulant administration; these, too, are considered negative responses. Careful assessment and documentation of the extent and course of responses to stimulant challenge are critical to the interpretation of its results and eventually, selection of therapeutic regimen.

Once TCA therapy is begun, plasma levels constitute a useful adjunct to clinical decision-making. Plasma levels are best described for nortriptyline and imipramine (Burrows & Norman, 1981). Nortriptyline demonstrates a therapeutic window; that is, plasma concentrations of 50–150 ng/ml are correlated with clinical therapeutic responses, whereas levels outside that range are not associated with significant clinical improvement (Friedel, 1982). Imipramine (Extein et al., 1984; Friedel, 1982), and perhaps the remainder of TCAs (Extein et al., 1984), show a sigmoidal relationship with therapeutic levels representing a threshold for clinical therapeutic response.

Many factors affect the validity and reliability of plasma TCA levels. For maximum accuracy, plasma levels must be drawn 10–12 hours after a patient has received the last dose (Friedel, 1982) although some protocols will accept blood samples taken after 8 hours (Gram et al., 1981). Accurate documentation of dosage and sampling times is essential for valid interpretation. Blood samples also need to be heparinized (Friedel, 1982) and cannot be taken in certain tubes, including vacutainers or others with rubber stoppers (Gram et al., 1981). Additional sources of significant error can be introduced by some specific methods of laboratory analysis (Extein et al., 1984; Gram et al., 1981). Various commercial preparations of a single TCA exhibit sufficient variability in biological activity to produce changes in TCA plasma levels that may not be correlated accurately with clinical course (Extein, et al., 1984). Finally, standardized plasma levels have been derived from data obtained from clearly defined research populations, usually having major depressive disorder with melancholia (Asberg, 1981). Plasma levels obtained from patients with mixed or uncertain diagnoses may not warrant the same interpretation.

Nonetheless, plasma TCA levels are useful in evaluating compliance (Friedel, 1982), toxic effects (Extein et al., 1984; Smith et al., 1980), and nonresponsive reactions (Bielski & Friedel, 1979; Zarifian & Rigal, 1982), all of which may necessitate changing therapeutic agents. In addition, plasma levels are of value in titrating dosages, especially in children or the elderly (Burrows & Norman, 1981; Extein et al., 1984; Friedel, 1982) whose dosage-response curves may not match standardized samples. Plasma levels may be unusually high if neuroleptics are administered concomitantly, (Nelson & Jatlow, 1980) or decreased if patients are using oral contraceptives, alcohol, barbiturates (Friedel, 1982), or smoking cigarettes (Extein et al., 1984). These require additional dose adjustments even after steady-state levels have been attained.

Despite this rapidly developing technology of biological measurements to guide therapeutic strategy, selection of specific TCA therapy remains a clinical judgment (Asberg, 1981; Extein et al., 1984), dependent on the accuracy with which clinical behaviors can be elicited and described. Nursing's responsibility in this regard cannot be overestimated. Thorough assessment of baseline information, followed by careful documentation of behavioral changes associated with affective disorder, as well as drug toxicity, is critical to successful clinical management of depressed patients.

Combination therapies.   The use of therapeutic combinations of anti-depressants with a host of other substances have proliferated both in response to the emergence of depressions refractory to traditional therapies and the expansion of biochemical models of affective disorders. Efficacy of these combinations in comparison to single-drug treatments remains largely untested (Moreines & Gold, 1984; Zarifian & Rigal, 1982) for methodological reasons. But one prospective study (White et al., 1980) did report equivalent improvement between single-drug and combination therapies without a concomitant significant increase in side effects for combination therapy. Most reviewers (Ananth & Luchins, 1977; Goldberg & Thorton, 1978; Moreines & Gold, 1984; Schuckit et al., 1971; Stern & Mendels, 1981; White & Simpson, 1981), impressed with the safety of current protocols and urgency of untreated depressions, recommend combination therapy for patients resistant to single-drug regimens.

Once safety considerations in the use of TCA–MAOI combinations were assured, protocols for these combinations quickly developed. Such a protocol (Goldberg & Thorton, 1978; Schuckit et al., 1971; Sethna, 1974; Spiker & Pugh, 1976) begins with a drug-free patient given TCA for three or more days followed by the addition of small doses of MAOI. Occasionally (Kline & Cooper, 1980; White & Simpson, 1981), TCA and MAOI can be started together in small dosages and cautiously increased. Dangerous hypertensive side-effects have resulted from the sequence of adding TCA to MAOI (Ananth & Luchins, 1977; Zarifian & Rigal, 1982) and, therefore, is not recommended. Careful assessment of clinical improvement, as well as for side effects, is a most significant contribution nurses can make to the progression of TCA–MAOI therapy in any individual case. Among common reactions are hypotension or hypertension, and, in previously unidentified bipolar patients, cycling into hypomanic states.

Lithium has antidepressant effects, not only for prophylaxis of recurrent episodes (Coppen & Abou-Saleh, 1983; Lydiard & Pearsall, 1984), but also in acute depressive syndromes (Ariele & Lepkifker, 1982; Mendels et al., 1972; Mendels et al., 1979), although its use as a single-agent antidepressant has been approved by the FDA only for bipolar depressions. Unipolar depressed patients most likely to respond to lithium are believed to have symptomatology similar to bipolar syndromes (Lydiard & Pearsall, 1984). Hypersomnia in a depressed individual is believed to predict positive lithium response either used alone (Friedel, 1976) or in combination with MAOIs (Hall, 1971; Himmelhoch et al.,

1972; Zall, 1971). Overall, however the depressive subpopulation most likely to respond to lithium remains poorly defined (Jefferson, 1983). Likewise efficacy studies have been poorly controlled, for the most part, or have other methodological defects (Stern & Mendels, 1981).

Nonetheless, protocols for combining lithium with TCAs (Lingjaerde et al., 1974) and MAOIs (Moreines & Gold, 1984; Zall, 1971) are currently available. In either case, it is generally recommended that the protocol begin with a patient having a relatively stable lithium level, then add the TCA or MAOI in very small doses (Moreines & Gold, 1984) to avoid cycling into a hypomanic episode. Careful evaluation for these changes once again constitutes a substantial nursing contribution to the titration of lithium combination protocols. If such a combination is designed for elderly patients, lower lithium dosages, more frequent plasma level monitoring, and careful evaluation of cardiovascular and renal status must be instituted (Jefferson, 1983), in addition to the usual evaluations needed to safely manage lithium alone (Jefferson & Griest, 1977; Johnson, 1980).

A variety of combinations using TCA or MAOI and a neurotransmitter precursor are also available. The most common of these is tryptophan, a serotonin percursor that is usually added in small amounts to MAOI (Coppen et al., 1963; Glassman & Platman, 1969; Moreines & Gold, 1984; Pare, 1963) or TCA (Shaw et al., 1972; Stern & Mendels, 1981). Efficacy of these combinations, especially with TCA, is questionable (Stern & Mendels, 1981) and combinations with MAOIs appear to give rise to significant side-effects, such as excessive drowsiness, nausea, and dizziness (Moreines & Gold, 1984). Other precursors such as DOPA, tyrosine, or 5-HTP have either failed to achieve adequate results, or are in very early clinical trials (Gelenberg et al., 1982).

The last of the combination drug therapies to be considered is that of stimulants and antidepressants. Few studies addressing issues of efficacy, target population, and likely mechanisms producing therapeutic results have been done, and those that do exist have been open trials with very small sample sizes. Nonetheless, several situations have been identified in which either dextroamphetamine or methylphenidate may be used in combination with antidepressants. The mood-elevating effects of amphetamines are well-known, short-lived, and subject to tolerance (Klerman, 1978). Yet, patients who respond positively to stimulant challenge tests may benefit from short-term (7–10 days) amphetamine or methylphenidate therapy until therapeutic results of TCA can develop. Discontinuation of the stimulant portion of the protocol needs to be gradual to avoid withdrawal effects. During the combination period, patients need to be assessed for the development of stimulant toxicity; equally as important is assessment for the occurence of hypomanic episodes in heretofore unrecognized bipolar patients. While this combination is not without its risks, the prompt alleviation of disabling depressive symptomatology speaks to the need to further investigate stimulant–antidepressant protocols.

Some symptom clusters found in depression also seem to respond to stimulant–antidepressive combinations. Depressions characterized by psychomotor retardation, even if occuring in the elderly (Katon & Raskind, 1980) or medically ill (Kaufmann & Murray, 1982), have improved promptly to stimulant therapy. Somewhat more surprising is the finding that elderly depressives with agitation also improved with amphetamine (Ward & Lampe, 1982). These combinations have not been used extensively enough to describe precise protocols for their use. It has also been suggested that methylphenidate may be a useful adjunct to TCA therapy to either increase plasma-TCA levels (Wharton et al., 1971) or to counteract postural hypotension (Flemenbaum, 1971), thereby increasing the likelihood that TCAs could have a therapeutic response. In both of these instances, a considerable amount of clinical judgment based on daily, or even hourly, assessments is required to use stimulant-TCA therapy.

Yet another combination strategy is available in the use of parenteral and oral TCAs. This strategy begins with parenteral TCA to raise plasma levels to therapeutic range, then uses oral TCA to maintain those levels (Bloomingdale & Bressler, 1979). In addition to being useful for patients who cannot or will not take oral medication initially, this protocol is intriguing because it shortens the length of time needed to achieve adequate plasma levels to 3 days (Ostow, 1974). Careful evaluation for cardiac arrhythmias is absolutely essential prior to beginning this treatment; some (Bloomingdale & Bressler, 1979) recommend skin-testing for TCA allergy. Blood-pressure measurements need to be a bit more frequent during the parenteral phase, but otherwise, nursing management is not significantly different from that of oral management.

Discussion of combination therapies would not be complete without some mention of anticholinergic reactions associated with antidepressants. Anticholinergic effects are well-documented (Cassem, 1982; Jefferson, 1975) and include dry mouth, constipation, and urinary retention. Indications of much more serious reactions are dilated pupils, tachycardia, flushing, dry skin, and the central effects of anxiety, delirium, disorientation, hyperactivity, and hallucinations (Granacher & Baldessarini, 1975). Combination therapies have a tendency to increase the likelihood of such anticholinergic reactions (Zarifian & Rigal, 1982). Intravenous physostigmine ordinarily produces prompt reversal of symptoms (Munoz, 1976), but may need to be repeated within 30 to 60 minutes due to the short-lived reaction of physostigmine (Bastani, 1979). Clearly, patients with acute anticholinergic reactions require precise clinical assessment and supportive care until they are safely stabilized. Such skilled care can be safely administered on psychiatric units if staff is adequately prepared to identify and respond to this physiological emergency.

Second generation antidepressants. Many new antidepressant substances are available either commercially or for clinical trials. Detailed descriptions of the substances and their activity are readily available (Ananth, 1983; Feighner, 1981; Feighner, 1983; Shopsin, 1980). Optimism about efficacy and safety of these highly specific medications makes them valuable adjuncts to current broad-spectrum therapies. However, the very newness of these drugs and the fact that their clinical trials have been limited to narrowly defined populations means that a considerable amount of clinical adjustment in suggested protocols is likely to be required to achieve safe, therapeutic responses. Nonetheless, these antidepressants represent yet another way in which antidepressant therapies are being successfully individualized for specific patient populations.

REFERENCES

Albala, A. A., Greden, J. F., Tarika, J., & Carroll, B. J. (1981). Changes in serial dexamethasone suppression tests among unipolar depressives receiving electroconvulsive treatment. *Biological Psychiatry, 16,* 551–560.

Ananth, J. (1983). New antidepressants. *Comprehensive Psychiatry, 24,* 116–124.

Ananth, J., & Luchins, D. (1977). A review of combined tricyclic and MAOI therapy. *Comprehensive Psychiatry, 18,* 221–230.

Arieli, A., & Lepkifker, E. (1981). The antidepressant effect of lithium. In W. B. Essman & L. Valzelli (Eds.), *Current developments in psychopharmacology, Vol. 6* (pp. 165–190). New York: Spectrum Publications.

Asberg, M. (1981). On the clinical importance of plasma concentrations of tricyclic antidepressant drugs. In E. Usdin (Ed.), *Clinical pharmacology in psychiatry* (pp. 301–309). New York: Elsevier.

Avery, D. H. & Winokur, G. (1977). The efficacy of electroconvulsive therapy and antidepressants in depression. *Biological Psychiatry, 12,* 507–523.

Bastani, J. R. (1979). Physostigmine treatment of tricyclic overdosage in psychosis. *Psychosomatics, 20,* 847–848.

Bates, B. A. (1983). *A guide to physical examination* (3rd ed.) (pp. 182–187). Philadelphia: J. B. Lippincott.

Bielski, R. J., & Friedel, R. O. (1979). Depressive subtypes defined by response to pharmacotherapy. *Psychiatric Clinics of North America, 2,* 483–497.

Bloomingdale, L. M. & Bressler, B. (1979). Rapid intramuscular administration of tricyclic antidepressants. *American Journal of Psychiatry, 136,* 1092–1093.

Brown, P., & Brawley, P. (1983). Dexamethasone suppression test and mood response to methylphenidate in primary depression. *American Journal of Psychiatry, 140,* 990–993.

Burrows, G. D., & Norman, T. R. (1981). Tricyclic antidepressants: Plasma levels and clinical response. In G. D. Burrows & T. R. Norman (Eds.), *Psychotropic drugs: Plasma concentration and clinical response* (pp. 169–204). New York: Marcel Dekker.

Carroll, B. J. (1982). Use of the dexamethasone suppression test in depression. *Journal of Clinical Psychiatry, 43,* (11, Sec. 2), 44–48.

Carroll, B. J. (1984). Dexamethasone suppression test for depression. In E. Usdin, M. Asberg, L. Bertilsson, & F. Sjoqvist (Eds.), *Frontiers in biochemical and pharmacological research in depression* (pp. 179–188). New York: Raven Press.

Carroll, B. J., Curtis, G. C., & Mendels, J. (1976). Neuroendocrine regulation in depression. II. Discrimination of depressed from nondepressed patients. *Archives of General Psychiatry, 33,* 1051–1058.

Cassem, J. (1982). Cardiovascular effects of antidepressants. *Journal of Clinical Psychiatry, 43,* 11(2), 22–28.

Coppen, A., & Abou-Saleh, M. T. (1983). Lithium in the prophylaxis of unipolar depression: A review. *Journal of the Royal Society of Medicine, 76,* 297–301.

Coppen, A., Shaw, D. M., & Farrell, J. P. (1963). Potentiation of the antidepressive effect of a monoamine oxidase inhibitor by tryptophan. *Lancet, 1,* 79–80.

Coryell, W. (1982). Hypothalamic–pituitary–adrenal axis abnormality and ECT response. *Psychiatry Research 6,* 283–292.

Davidson, J., McCeod, M. N., & Blum, M. R. (1978). Acetylation phenotype, platelet monoamine oxidase inhibition, and the effectiveness of phenelzine in depression. *American Journal of Psychiatry, 135,* 467–469.

Davis, J. (1976). Overview: Maintenance therapy in psychiatry: II. Affective disorders. *American Journal of Psychiatry, 133,* 1–13.

Ettigi, P. G., Hayes, P. E., Narasimhachari, N., Hamer, R. M., Goldberg, S., & Secord, G. J. (1983). D-amphetamine response and dexamethasone suppression test as predictors of treatment outcomes in unipolar depression. *Biological Psychiatry, 18,* 499–504.

Extein, I., Pottash, A. L. C., Gold, M. S., Goggans, R., & Lydiard, R. B. (1984). Antidepressants: Predicting response/maximizing efficacy. In M. S. Gold, R. B. Lydiard, & J. S. Carman (Eds.), *Advances in psychopharmacology: Predicting and improving treatment response* (pp. 83–106). Boca Raton, FL: CRC Press.

Fawcett, J., & Siomopoulos, V. (1971). Dextroamphetamine response as a possible predictor of improvement with tricyclic therapy in depression. *Archives of General Psychiatry, 25,* 247–255.

Fawcett, J., Maas, J. W., & Dekirmenjian, H. (1972). Depression and MHPG excretion. *Archives of General Psychiatry, 26,* 246–251.

Feighner, J. P. (1981). Clinical efficacy of the newer antidepressants. *Journal of Clinical Psychopharmacology, 1,* (6 Suppl.), 23–26.

Feighner, J. P. (1983). The new generation of antidepressants. *Journal of Clinical Psychiatry, 44* (5 Sec. 2), 49–55.

Fink, M. A. (1978). Efficacy and safety of induced seizures (EST) in man. *Comprehensive Psychiatry, 19,* 1–18.

Flemenbaum, A. (1971). Methylphenidate: A catalyst for the tricyclic antidepressants? *American Journal of Psychiatry, 128,* 239–240.

Fraser, A. R. (1983). Choice of antidepressant based on the dexamethasone suppression test. *American Journal of Psychiatry, 140,* 786–787.

Friedel, R. O. (1976). Lithium and depression. *American Journal of Psychiatry, 133,* 976–981.

Friedel, R. O. (1982). The relationship of therapeutic response to antidepressant plasma levels: An update. *Journal of Clinical Psychiatry, 43,* 11(2), 37–42.

Gelenberg, A. J., Gibson, C. J., & Wojcik, J. D. (1982). Neurotransmitter precursors for the treatment of depression. *Psychopharmacology Bulletin, 18,* 7–18.

Glassman, A. H., Giardina, E. V., Perel, J. M., Bigger, J. T., Kantor, S. J., & Davies,

M. (1979). Clinical characteristics of imipramine-induced orthostatic hypotension. *Lancet, 1,* 468–472.

Glassman, A., & Platman, S. (1969). Potentiation of a monoamine oxidase inhibitor by tryptophan. *Journal of Psychiatric Research, 7,* 83–85.

Goldberg, R. S., & Thorton, W. E. (1978). Combined tricyclic-MAOI therapy for refractory depression: A review, with guidelines for appropriate usage. *Journal of Clinical Pharmacology, 18,* 143–147.

Gram, L. F., Bech, P., Reisby, N., & Jorgenson, O. S. (1981). Methodology in studies on plasma level/effect relationship of tricyclic antidepressants. In E. Usdin (Ed.), *Clinical pharmacology in psychiatry* (pp. 155–171). New York: Elsevier.

Granacher, R. P., & Baldessarini, R. P. (175). Physostigmine. *Archives of General Psychiatry, 32,* 375–380.

Hall, H. (1971). Lithium and isocarboxazid, an effective drug approach to severe depressions. *American Journal of Psychiatry, 127,* 1400–1401.

Heninger, G. R., Charney, D. S., & Menkes, D. B. (1983). Receptor sensitivity and the mechanism of action of antidepressant treatment. In P. J. Clayton & J. E. Barrett (Eds.), *Treatment of depression: Old controversies and new approaches* (pp. 133–151). New York: Raven Press.

Himmelhoch, J. M., Detre, T., Kupfer, D. J., Swartzsburg, M., & Byck, R. (1972). Treatment of previously intractable depressions with tranylcypromine and lithium. *Journal of Nervous and Mental Diseases, 155,* 216–220.

Jefferson, J. W. (1975). A review of the cardiovascular effects and toxicity of tricyclic antidepressants. *Psychosomatic Medicine, 37,* 160–179.

Jefferson, J. W. (1983). Lithium and affective disorder in the elderly. *Comprehensive Psychiatry, 124,* 166–178.

Jefferson, J. W., & Griest, J. H. (1977). *Primer of lithium therapy.* Baltimore: Williams & Wilkins.

Johnson, F. N. (Ed.). (1980). *Handbook of lithium therapy.* Lancaster, PA: MTP Press.

Katon, W., Raskind, M. (1980). Treatment of depression in the medically ill elderly with methylphenidate. *American Journal of Psychiatry, 137,* 963–965.

Kaufmann, M. W., & Murray, G. B. (1982). The use of d-amphetamine in medically ill depressed patients. *Journal of Clinical Psychiatry, 43,* 463–464.

Kiloh, L. G., Neilson, M., & Andrews, G. (1974). Response of depressed patients to methylamphetamine. *British Journal of Psychiatry, 125,* 496–499.

Klein, D. F., Gittelman, R., Quitkin, F., & Rifkin, A. (1980). *Diagnosis and drug treatment of psychiatric disorders: Adults and children (2nd ed.)* (pp. 449–492). Baltimore: Williams & Wilkins.

Klerman, G. L. (1978). Psychopharmacologic treatment of depression. In J. G. Bernstein (Ed.), *Clinical Pharmacology* (pp. 63–79). Littleton, MA: PSG Publishing.

Kline, N. S. & Cooper, T. B. (1980). Monoamine oxidase in inhibitors as antidepressants. In F. Hoffmeister & G. Stille (Eds.), *Psychotropic agents, Part I. Antipsychotics and antidepressants* (pp. 369–397). New York: Springer/Verlag.

Lingjaerde, O., Edlund, A. H., Gormsen, C. A., Gottfries, C. G., Haugstad, A., Hermann, I. L., Hollnagel, P., Makimattilla, A., Rassmussen, K. E., Remvig, J., & Robak, O. H. (1974). The effects of lithium carbonate in combination with tricyclic antidepressants in endogenous depression. A double-blind, multicenter trial. *Acta Psychiatrica Scandinavica, 50,* 233–242.

Lydiard, R. B., & Pearsall, R. (1984). Lithium: Predicting response/maximizing efficacy. In M. S. Gold, R. B. Lydiard, & J. S. Carman (Eds.), *Advances in psychopharmacology: Predicting and improving treatment response* (pp. 121–155). Boca Raton, FL: CRC Press.

Maas, J. W., Fawcett, J. A., & Dekirmenjian, H. (1972). Catecholamine metabolism, depressive illness and drug response. *Archives of General Psychiatry, 26,* 252–262.

Mendels, J., Ramsey, A., Dyson, W. & Fraser, A. (1979). Lithium as an antidepressant. *Archives of General Psychiatry, 36,* 845–851.

Mendels, J., Secunda, S. K., & Dyson, W. L. (1972). A controlled study of the antidepressant effects of lithium. *Archives of General Psychiatry, 26,* 154–157.

Moreines, R., & Gold, M. S. (1984). MAOInhibitors: Predicting response/maximizing efficacy. In M. S. Gold, R. B. Lydiard, & J. S. Carman (Eds.), *Advances in psychopharmacology: Predicting and improving treatment response* (pp. 157–177). Boca Raton, FL: CRC Press.

Morris, J. B., & Beck, A. T. (1974). The efficacy of antidepressant drugs. *Archives of General Psychiatry, 30,* 667–676.

Munoz, R. A. (1976). Treatment of tricyclic intoxication. *American Journal of Psychiatry, 133,* 1085–1087.

Nelson, J. C., & Jatlow, P. I. (1980). Neuroleptic effect on desipramine steady-state plasma concentrations. *American Journal of Psychiatry, 137,* 1232–1234.

Oswald, I., Brezinova, V., & Dunleavy, D. F. (1972). On the slowness of action of tricyclic antidepressant drugs. *British Journal of Psychiatry, 120,* 673–677.

Ostow, M. (1974). Rapid and gentle pharmacotherapy of depression. *New York State Journal of Medicine, 1,* 74–77.

Pare, C. (1963). Potentiation of momoamine oxidase inhibitors by tryptophan. *Lancet, 2,* 527–528.

Preskorn, S. H., & Irwin, H. A. (1982). Toxicity of tricyclic antidepressants—kinetics, mechanism, intervention: A review. *Journal of Clinical Psychiatry, 43,* 151–156.

Raft, D., Davison, J., Wasik, J., & Mattox, A. (1981). Relationship between response to phenelzine and MAO inhibition in a clinical trial of phenelzine, amitriptyline and placebo. *Neuropsychobiology, 7,* 122–125.

Ravaris, C., Nies, A., Robinson, D., Ives, J., Lamborn, K., & Korson, L. (1976). A multiple-dose, controlled study of phenelzine in depression-anxiety states. *Archives of General Psychiatry, 33,* 347–349.

Richelson, E. (1982). Pharmacology of antidepressants in use in the United States. *Journal of Clinical Psychiatry, 43,* 11(2), 4–11.

Robinson, D. S., Nies, A., Ravaris, C. L., & Lambourn, K. R. (1973). The monoamine oxidase inhibitor phenelzine in the treatment of depressive anxiety states. *Archives of General Psychiatry, 29,* 407–413.

Robinson, D., Nies, A., Ravaris, C., Ives, J., & Bartlett, D. (1978). Clinical pharmacology of phenelzine. *Archives of General Psychiatry, 35,* 629–631.

Sabelli, H. C. & Mosnaim, A. D. (1974). Phenylethylamine hypothesis of affective behavior. *American Journal of Psychiatry, 131,* 695–699.

Sabelli, H. C., Fawcett, J., Gusovsky, F., Javaid, J., Edwards, J., & Jeffries, H. (1983a). Urinary phenyl acetate: A diagnostic test for depression? *Science, 220,* 1187–1188.

Sabelli, H. C., Fawcett, J., Javaid, J. I., & Bagri, S. (1983b). The methylphenidate test for differentiating desipramine-responsive from nortriptyline-responsive depression. *American Journal of Psychiatry, 140,* 212–214.

Schoonover, S. C. (1983). Depression. In E. L. Bassuk, S. C. Schoonover, & A. J. Gelenberg (Eds.), *The practitioner's guid to psychoactive drugs* (2nd ed.) (pp. 19–77). New York: Plenum Medical Books.

Schuckit, M., Robins, E., & Geighner, J. (1971). Tricyclic antidepressants and mono-amine oxidase inhibitors. Combination therapy in the treatment of depression. *Archives of General Psychiatry, 24,* 509–514.

Sethna, E. R. (1974) A study of refractory cases of depressive illnesses and their response to combined antidepressant treatment. *British Journal of Psychiatry,* 124, 265–272.

Shaw, D. M., Johnson, A. L., & MacSweeney, D. A. (1972). Tricyclic antidepressants and tryptophan in unipolar affective disorder. *Lancet, 2,* 1245–1246.

Shopsin, B. (1980). Second generation antidepressants. *Journal of Clinical Psychiatry, 41,* 12(2), 45–56.

Shopsin, B., & Kline, N. S. (1976). Monoamine oxidase inhibitors: Potential for drug abuse. *Biological Psychiatry, 11,* 451–456.

Smith, R. C., Chojnacki, M., Hu, R., & Mann, E. (1980). Cardiovascular effects of therapeutic doses of tricyclic antidepressants: Importance of blood level monitoring. *Journal of Clinical Psychiatry, 41,* 12(2), 57–63.

Spiker, D. G. & Pugh, D. D. (1976). Combining tricyclic and monoamine oxidase inhibitor antidepressants. *Archives of General Psychiatry, 33,* 828–830.

Stern, S. L., & Mendels, J. (1981). Drug combinations in the treatment of refractory depression: A review. *Journal of Clinical Psychiatry, 42,* 368–373.

Stern, S. L., Rush, A. J., & Mendels, J. (1980). Toward a rational pharmacotherapy of depression. *American Journal of Psychiatry, 135,* 545–552.

Van Kammen, D. P., & Murphy, D. L. (1978). Prediction of imipramine response by a one-day d-amphetamine trial. *American Journal of Psychiatry, 135,* 1179–1184.

Ward, N. G., & Lampe, T. H. (1982). A trial of dextroamphetamine in patients with involutional agitated depression. *Journal of Clinical Psychiatry, 43,* 35–36.

Wharton, R. N., Perel, J. M., & Dayton, P. G. (1971). A potential clinical use for methylphenidate with tricyclic antidepressants. *American Journal of Psychiatry, 127,* 1619–1625.

White, K., Pistole, T., & Boyd, J. (1980). Combined monoamine oxidase inhibitor-tricyclic antidepressant treatment: A pilot study. *American Journal of Psychiatry, 137,* 1422–1424.

White, K., & Simpson, G. (1981). Combined MAOI-tricyclic antidepressant treatment: A reevaluation. *Journal of Clinical Psychopharmacology, 1,* 164–169.

Zall, H. (1971). Lithium carbonate and isocarboxazid—an effective drug approach in severe depressions. *American Journal of Psychiatry, 127,* 1400–1403.

Zarifian, E., & Rigal, F. (1982). New antidepressants and trends in the pharmacotherapy of depressive disorders. *Psychiatric Clinics of North America, 6,* 129–139.

Index

A

Abnormal (diminished) GH secretion, 25
Acetylcholine in current research, 20, 27
ACTH. *See* Adrenocorticotropic hormone
Acute mania. *See* Mania
Acute organic brain syndrome as adverse
    affect of ECT-induced therapy,
    96
Adjustment, support or maintenance
    levels of, nursing interventions
    for, 134–135(*t*), 136
Adrenocorticotropic hormone (ACTH) in
    current research, 22–23
Affective disorders, biochemical theories
    of. *See* Biochemical theories of
    affective disorders
Affective illness, current research in
  biogenic hypothesis in, 15
  brain imaging in, 29
  catecholamine hypothesis in, 16–17
  diagnostic issues in, 14–15
  growth hormone and, 25
  indoleamine hypothesis in, 18
  LHPA in, 22–24
  LHPT in, 24–25
  lithium transport in, 28–29

neuroendocrine hypothesis in, 22
  phenylethylamine hypothesis in, 18–19
  stimulant challenge test in, 26–28
  two-amine hypothesis in, 19–20
Aggression of depressed child, specific
    interventions for, 174–175
Alcohol abuse as cause of depression,
    209
Alpha-para-tyrosine (AMPT) in current
    research, 17
AMI. *See* Amitriptylene
Amitriptylene (AMI) in current research,
    17, 20, 21, 27
Amnesia, 94–95
Amphetamines
  as used in combination with
    stimulants, 228, 229. *See also*
    Antidepressant therapies, use of
    therapeutic combinations of
  in current research, 25
AMPT. *See* Alpha-methyl-para-tyrosine
Anaclitic depression, 162
Anger, arousal of as indicator of clinical
    improvement, 92
Anhedonia, as symptom of depression,
    56, 57
Anterograde amnesia, 95